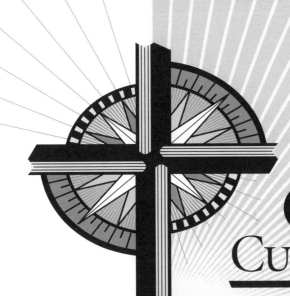

CONCORDIA
CURRICULUM GUIDE

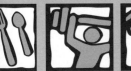   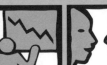

GRADE
6

Health

CONCORDIA PUBLISHING HOUSE • SAINT LOUIS

Copyright © 2007 Concordia Publishing House
3558 S. Jefferson Ave., St. Louis, MO 63118-3968
1-800-325-3040 • www.cph.org

Prepared with materials provided by Vicki Boye and Jacalyn Schulze

Edited by Clarence Berndt

Series editors: Carolyn Bergt, Clarence Berndt, and Rodney L. Rathmann

This publication may be available in braille, in large print, or on cassette tape for the visually impaired. Please allow 8 to 12 weeks for delivery. Write to the Library for the Blind, 7550 Watson Rd., St. Louis, MO 63119-4409; call toll-free 1-888-215-2455; or visit the Web site: www.blindmission.org.

Manufactured in the United States of America

CONTENTS

PREFACE

The Ministry of Christian Schools

Parents expect Christian schools to provide excellent discipline, meet high academic standards, have low teacher-student ratios, and be staffed by dedicated, conscientious teachers. Many schools meet these expectations, but the distinguishing feature of a Christian school is that the school proclaims Jesus Christ to be the Son of God and Savior of the world. Teaching Jesus Christ, then, is the real difference between Christian and public schools. In Christian schools, teachers and students witness personally and publicly to their faith in Jesus Christ. Students study the Bible and worship God daily. Teachers relate Jesus Christ to all aspects of the curriculum. Teachers and students share Christian love and forgiveness.

Those who teach in Lutheran schools have the privilege and opportunity to

- teach the Word of God in its truth and purity;

- acknowledge the Bible as God's infallible Word and the Confessions as the true exposition of the Word;

- identify God's Word, Baptism, and the Lord's Supper as the means through which God creates and sustains faith;

- emphasize Law and Gospel as the key teachings of Scripture;

- apply Law and Gospel properly in daily relationships with students, parents, and other teachers;

- teach all of what Scripture teaches (including Christian doctrines) to all students, no matter what backgrounds they have;

- share with students what Jesus the Savior means to them personally;

- equip students to proclaim the Good News;

- provide students the support and encouragement found only in the body of Christ, of which Jesus Himself is the head.

In Christian schools, Christ permeates all subjects and activities. Religion is not limited to one hour or one class. Teachers seek opportunities to witness in every class and to relate God's Word to all aspects of life. Through this process, and by the power of the Holy Spirit, students grow in faith and in a sanctified life, and view all of life, not just Sunday, as a time to serve and worship God. It is intrinsic to ministry in a Christian school that all energies expended in the educational process lead each child to a closer relationship with the Savior and with other members of the Christian community.

How to Use This Guide

The Concordia Curriculum Guide (CCG) series is designed to guide you as you plan and prepare to teach. The introductory chapters provide foundational information relevant to teaching health in a Christian school, but the majority of the pages in this volume focus on health standards and performance expectations together with ideas and activities for integrating them with various aspects of the Christian faith. This volume is not intended to provide a curriculum plan or lesson plan for any particular period or day. Instead, it provides a wealth of ideas from which you can choose and a springboard to new ideas you may create. You may use this curriculum guide with any set of health materials.

The health standards included in this book are informed by the standards developed by the American Association for Health Education (AAHE), in cooperation with the American Cancer Society (see also Chapter 3) and are provided as a compilation of the health standards and performance expectations adopted by the individual states. In order to offer a well-coordinated curriculum design, the health objectives for this grade level relate to and connect with the standards provided at other grade levels.

The Concordia Health Standards, then, can serve you and your faculty in several ways. They can help you

1. plan your teaching in an organized way;

2. coordinate your teaching of health with health teaching in other grades in your school;

3. select textbooks and other learning or teaching materials that help your students excel in meeting standards in health education;

4. evaluate your current health policies, instruction, materials, and objectives;

5. implement procedures for school accreditation;

6. nurture the Christian faith of your students as you teach health concepts and practices.

We assume that teachers will use materials in addition to those included in the guide, but, since many materials do not relate health education to the Christian faith, we have provided suggestions for specific faith connections to use as you teach day after day. Additionally, we know that everyone has a different teaching style. No one will be able to use all the ideas in this volume. As you think about practices that will work for you and would be helpful in your classroom, consider these possible ways to find and use ideas from this volume:

- Read the entire volume before the school year begins. Highlight the ideas you want to use.

- Write ideas or references to this volume in your textbooks or other health teaching materials. List the page and standard numbers from this volume that contain suggestions you would like to use in connection with a lesson or unit.

- Designate periods of time throughout the year, perhaps at faculty meetings, to discuss portions of this volume as you, along with fellow staff members, seek to improve your integration of the faith in health education activities. Brainstorm, develop, and implement your ideas. Share your successes and challenges in subsequent meetings. Together, find ways to effectively use the suggestions in this Concordia Curriculum Guide volume.

- Plan ways to adapt ideas in the CCG health volumes that are not closely related to specific lessons or units in your textbooks. Inside your plan book, clip a list of suggestions from the volume that you would like to use, or list each idea on a file card and keep the cards handy for quick review. Use those ideas between units or when extra time is available.

- Evaluate each suggestion after you have tried it. Label it as "use again" or "need to revise." Always adapt the suggestions to fit your situation.

- Think about how you might nurture the faith of students each time you plan a health lesson. Set a goal for yourself (e.g., two ideas from this volume each week), and pray that God will help you to achieve it. You will find the index of this volume helpful in finding faith-connecting activities related to specific topics.

- If the ideas in the Concordia Curriculum Guide series seem overwhelming, begin by concentrating on only one subject per month, or attempt to use the suggested ideas in only two to four subjects the first year. Add two to four subjects per year after that.

Probably the most effective teaching occurs when teachers take advantage of natural opportunities that arise to integrate the faith into their teaching. In those situations you will often use your own ideas instead of preparing a lesson plan based on teaching suggestions in this guide. Use the white space on the pages of this book to record your own ideas and activities for integrating the Christian faith into your health lessons. We hope this volume will be an incentive to you to create your own effective ways to integrate the Christian faith into the entire school day. We believe that Christian schools are essential because we believe that our relationship with Jesus Christ is essential to eternal life. Nurturing the faith in children must permeate every part of our lives and all aspects of Christian education. That is why our Christian faith permeates our teaching. That is why we teach in a Christian school.

CHAPTER 1

Health Education in the Christian School

Vicki Boye

Vicki L. Boye, PhD, is Associate Professor of Health and Human Performance and a graduate of Concordia University Nebraska. She did her graduate work at the University of Houston (MS, 1989) and earned a doctorate from the University of Nebraska in health education (1999). She has taught at Lutheran high schools in Kansas City and Houston. While at Lutheran High North in Houston, she was named Teacher of the Year in 1989. Currently, her primary responsibilities are in the areas of health education and lifetime wellness. She has written for *Lutheran Education*, is a member of the CUS Council for Physical Activity and Wellness, and provides health seminars and presentations to various community and campus groups.

Health and Wellness: A Holistic Approach

Health is more than the absence of disease; it is more than one's physical condition or state, as has been the traditional idea. Health is multi-dimensional and dynamic in nature. Health is defined as the state or quality of one's spiritual, physical, emotional, career (occupational), intellectual, environmental, and social well-being. Wellness is defined as the ongoing and deliberate effort to achieve and maintain one's optimal level of these factors (Hoeger and Hoeger 2007). These seven interrelated dimensions or components of health and wellness may more easily be remembered by using the acronym SPECIES. Health and wellness encompass the human SPECIES and health education embraces each of these dimensions.

Spiritual: The underlying foundation for all other dimensions, it is the recognition of and faith in our Lord and Savior, Jesus Christ (i.e., having a relationship and being "right" with our loving God). Lutheran educators teach God's Word to nurture faith in the Lord Jesus within young people. God's Word provides a motivation for a sanctified life as it guides the children of God in their morals, values, and ethics.

Physical: Proper structure and function of body systems, absence or minimal impact from disease/disorders or disabilities, ability to perform daily tasks without undue fatigue and with proper health and nutrition habits. In this dimension,

health education teachers provide instruction about the continuing care of the blessings God has given us as He created us.

Emotional: The ability to understand and express developmentally appropriate emotions as well as achieve and maintain emotional stability. In the emotional dimension, teachers help students recognize and understand their feelings as well as develop the ability to express these emotions in appropriate ways.

Career (Occupational): The ability to effectively perform and develop satisfaction, fulfillment, and a sense of self-worth in one's work. In this dimension, teachers encourage students to effectively meet the demands and challenges of their vocation in the present time, as well as the future, doing all to the glory of God.

Intellectual: The ability to think and process information at a developmentally appropriate level. Teachers cultivate the joy of learning through this dimension, providing opportunities for students to learn and engage in developmentally appropriate reflection and activity.

Environmental: The recognition and acceptance of one's place and responsibility as a member of God's creation. In the environmental dimension, teachers nurture their students' appreciation and respect for the environment, encouraging them to embrace their responsibility as faithful stewards of God's creation.

Social: The ability to interact with others and develop and maintain relationships. In this dimension, teachers help students develop their intrapersonal and interpersonal skills in positive ways, to aid in forming and sustaining healthful relationships.

Knowledge, Skills, and Attitudes

The purpose of health education, whether in school, at home, or in the community, is to (a) increase positive health behaviors, and (b) reduce health risk behaviors. In order to influence behaviors, health educators must take a triadic approach that involves the development of students' knowledge, skills, and attitudes. *Knowledge* encompasses the cognitive domain—the comprehension of health facts and concepts. *Skills* are the abilities and tools students need to effectively deal with life experiences in a healthy manner. (These include not only physical skills, such as brushing one's teeth properly, but also social and life skills such as decision-making, problem-solving, and communication skills—all of which are needed to live an abundant life.) *Attitudes* refer to the values, morals, and beliefs that guide students' decisions and life choices.

In the past, health education programs have been heavily knowledge-based in nature. However, to truly foster healthy behaviors, knowledge, skills, and attitudes must be equally addressed and incorporated into the health curriculum. As teachers in a Christian school we have the opportunity and privilege to teach not only the *how* with respect to healthy behaviors but also the all-important *why*—because we have been redeemed by Christ Jesus and Him crucified.

Comprehensive Health Education

According to the Centers for Disease Control's Healthy Youth program, the following are key elements of a comprehensive health education program:

• A documented, planned, and sequential program of health instruction for students in grades kindergarten through twelve.

• A curriculum that addresses and integrates education about a range of categorical health problems and issues at developmentally appropriate ages.

• Activities that help young people develop the skills they need to avoid tobacco use; dietary patterns that contribute to disease; sedentary lifestyle; sexual behaviors that result in HIV infection, other STDs, and unintended pregnancy; alcohol and other drug use; and behaviors that result in unintentional and intentional injuries.

• Instruction provided for a prescribed amount of time at each grade level.

• Management and coordination by an education professional trained to implement the program.

• Instruction from teachers who are trained to teach the subject.

• Involvement of parents, health professionals, and other concerned community members.

• Periodic evaluation, updating, and improvement.

Source: www.cdc.gov/HealthyYouth/CSHP/comprehensive_ed.htm

One Piece of the Puzzle

Comprehensive health education is but one piece of the puzzle in the school's effort to establish and maintain a coordinated school health program "designed to protect, promote, and improve the health and well-being of students and staff, thus improving a student's ability to learn" (Joint Terminology Committee, 2001, p. 99). According to the National Association of State Boards of Education, an effective coordinated school health program involves the following eight unique, yet interrelated, components:

• A school environment that is safe and that physically, socially, and psychologically promotes health-enhancing behaviors.

• A sequential health education curriculum that is designed to motivate and help students maintain and improve their health, prevent disease, and avoid health-related risk behaviors.

- A sequential physical education curriculum that involves moderate to vigorous physical activity; teaches knowledge, motor skills, and positive attitudes; and promotes activities and sports that all students enjoy and can pursue throughout their lives.

- A nutrition program that includes a food service program that serves appealing choices of nutritious foods; a sequential program of nutrition instruction that is integrated within the comprehensive school health education curriculum; and a school environment that encourages students to make healthy food choices.

- A school health services program that is designed to ensure access or referral to primary health-care services, prevent and control communicable disease and other health problems, and provide emergency care for illness or injury provided by well-qualified and well-supported health professionals.

- A counseling, psychological, and social services program that is designed to ensure access or referral to assessments, interventions, and other mental, emotional, and social health services for students.

- Integrated family and community involvement activities that are designed to engage families as active participants in their children's education and that encourage collaboration with community resources and services to respond more effectively to the health-related needs of students.

- A health promotion program that provides opportunities for school staff to improve their health status through activities such as health assessments, health education, and health-related fitness activities.

For more information go to www.nasbe.org/healthy_schools/intro.htm.

Our Responsibility as Christian Educators

As children of God and teachers who serve God's people, we have the responsibility and duty to tend to the needs of Lutheran school families in all seven dimensions of health (Spiritual, Physical, Emotional, Career/Occupational, Intellectual, Environmental, and Social). From diseases (Exodus 4:6; Luke 16:20) and risky behaviors (Romans 13:13; Proverbs 23:21) to coping with stress (Psalm 55:22) and social relationships (1 Thessalonians 5:12–14), along with other issues, God guides us through His Word. Use the Scriptures as a resource as you work to provide your students with the knowledge, skills, and attitudes to live long, healthy, God-pleasing lives, honoring Him with their bodies, minds, and spirits with which He has blessed them.

Not only has God blessed us with a wonderful body, He has redeemed it through the life, death, and resurrection of His only Son, who came from heaven to take our human form upon Himself. Now, by faith, He equips and empowers us to honor Him in the new and eternal life He has given us to live for Him. Reflect on the implications of this new life for the body God has given us with this verse from 1 Corinthians: "Do you not know that your body is a temple of the Holy Spirit within you, whom you have from God? You are not your own, for you were bought with a price. So glorify God in your body" (6:19–20).

References

Centers for Disease Control. Healthy Youth: Coordinated School Health Program. 2006. http://www.cdc.gov/HealthyYouth/CSHP/ (accessed May 15, 2006).

Hoeger, W. and Hoeger, S., *Lifetime Physical Fitness and Wellness*, (Ninth Edition), (Belmont, CA: Thomson Wadsworth, 2007).

Joint Committee on Health Education and Health Promotion Terminology. 2001. Report of the 2000 Joint Committee on Health Education and Health Promotion Terminology. *Journal of Health Education* 61 (2): 89–103.

National Association of State Boards of Education. 2006. Healthy Schools: Sample General School Health Policies. http://www.nasbe.org/HealthySchools/Health_Policies.html (accessed May 15, 2006).

CHAPTER 2

Teaching and Learning about Personal Health from a Christian Perspective

By faith Christians know that God "provides all that we need to sustain this body and life." In His great love, He sustains and upholds us even as He has sent His only Son to redeem all people. Humans are the highest of God's creation, the focus of His redeeming love in Jesus Christ, and the objects of the Holy Spirit's nurturing work. In response to His care for us, body and soul, our bodies deserve our most excellent respect.

Health information and all other subjects can be taught and learned through the following overall goals, which have been the hallmark of the Christian education material prepared by Concordia Publishing House through the years and are the hallmark of the Concordia Curriculum Guide series. These materials aim to assist teachers and leaders so that

- through the Word of God and the work of the Holy Spirit, people of all ages may know God, especially His seeking and forgiving love in Christ, and may respond in faith and grow into Christian maturity;

- seeing themselves as the reconciled, redeemed children of God and individual members of Christ's body, the Church, students may live in peace with God, themselves, and their fellow human beings;

- students may be encouraged to express their joy when they worship God and when they give loving service to others;

- by the grace of God, students may value all of God's creative work in His world, witness openly to Christ as the Savior of all people, and participate actively in God's mission to the Church and the world;

- students may joyfully live in the Christian hope of new life in Christ now and in eternity.

Personal Health and God

Our loving and almighty God cares for us and is concerned about our every bodily need. Above all, He loves and desires to save all people through faith in Jesus Christ. Any course of instruction about understanding and caring for our health and well-being that ignores the Creator and Preserver of all things is incomplete.

For the children of God, learning good health practices involves knowledge and understanding of the following:

- God is the creator of our bodies and is the one who saves and provides for us.

- We are the receivers and stewards of God's gift of the human body.

- Nonbelievers are also God's creation and are to be stewards of this gift as well.

- All creation is God's gift for the preservation and support of human life.

God's Word teaches these truths:

- God created our first parents, Adam and Eve, and through them all people.

- Yielding to the temptation to abandon God's will, Adam and Eve sinned. All of creation, including the human body, suffered sin's devastating consequences.

- Although God made people in His image, that image was lost by our first parents; through the fall into sin it is lost in all people who come after them (Genesis 5:3).

- The ravages of sin and our separation from God are still evident in our bodies and in all creation (Genesis 3).

- God sent His only Son to live, die, and rise again in order to pay for the sins of all people (2 Corinthians 5:15). Jesus is the Son of God and also true man; He is fully and truly divine and fully and truly human. Salvation can be found only in Him (Acts 4:12).

- As God who created all things, Jesus exerts control over the forces of nature as they affect our bodies. For example, He healed many people (e.g., Matthew 12:13 and Mark 6:56), and He reversed the natural decaying process when He raised Lazarus from the dead (John 11:38–44).

- As true man, Jesus understands what it means to be human. He knew hunger and fatigue, humiliation and pain, compassion and amazement, friendship and joy. He has been tempted in every way, just as we are—yet was without sin (Hebrews 4:15).

- Jesus used His body to accomplish our salvation. Taking our sin and punishment upon Himself, Jesus overcame even His own death, rising from the dead on Easter morning (Matthew 28:6–7). Through His life, death, and resurrection, Jesus earned forgiveness for all our sin and provides us with a new and eternal life in His name (2 Corinthians 5:17).

- It is God's desire that all people come to faith in Jesus and receive the forgiveness, new life, and salvation He offers freely in Christ Jesus (1 Timothy 2:4). God wants His Word and the Sacraments administered faithfully so that all people may come to believe in Him and be saved (2 Peter 3:9).

Health Education and Ourselves

Any comprehension of the human experience must begin with a basic understanding of the value God places on the individual. Although we are sinful from birth, God sent His Son, Jesus, to buy us back from sin, death, and Satan's power. This sacrificial love indicates God's great love for each person. The psalmist David worshiped God for the goodness He extended to him as a human being: "Bless the LORD, O my soul, and forget not all His benefits, who forgives all your iniquity, who heals all your diseases, who redeems your life from the pit, who crowns you with steadfast love and mercy, who satisfies you with good so

that your youth is renewed like the eagle's" (Psalm 103:2–5). Paul tells us that God values every human being, you included. "You were bought with a price. So glorify God in your body" (1 Corinthians 6:20).

God's Word teaches these truths:

- God the Holy Spirit brings us to faith through the power of God's Word.

- God's faithful people respond to the Gospel of Jesus Christ with lives that demonstrate Christ's love (1 Thessalonians 2:13).

- God knows each of us by name. Isaiah records, "Fear not, for I have redeemed you; I have called you by name, you are Mine" (Isaiah 43:1). He further knows all about us, including the designations we will have throughout our life that identify us according to our profession, hobbies and interests, religious denomination, and political affiliation.

- Each person is important to God. Matthew writes, "Are not two sparrows sold for a penny? And not one of them will fall to the ground apart from your Father. But even the hairs of your head are all numbered. Fear not, therefore; you are of more value than many sparrows" (Matthew 10:29–31). God knows all our personality quirks and inconsistencies. In His Word and Sacraments, He remains with us to guide and direct us through the twists and turns of our lives.

- God knows us better than anyone else knows us. He knows us better than we know ourselves. Of God, the psalmist writes, "For You formed my inward parts; You knitted me together in my mother's womb. I praise You, for I am fearfully and wonderfully made. Wonderful are Your works; my soul knows it very well. My frame was not hidden from You, when I was being made in secret, intricately woven in the depths of the earth. Your eyes saw my unformed substance; in Your book were written, every one of them, the days that were formed for me, when as yet there were none of them" (Psalm 139:13–16).

- God has a plan for each human life. He made us individually and with unique qualities, aptitudes, and interests. He helps those who belong to Him through faith in Christ Jesus to serve Him in every aspect of life. "For I know the plans I have for you, declares the LORD, plans for wholeness and not for evil, to give you a future and a hope" (Jeremiah 29:11). His Spirit empowers us to serve Him in our life's roles and vocations, whatever they may be.

- God treasures every human being and sent His Son to redeem all people, even those with developmental disabilities and other bodily conditions, whatever they might be. In response to Christ's love for all people, He calls us to honor and respect others, to "help and support him in every physical need," and to "defend him, speak well of him, and explain everything in the kindest possible way" (explanations of the Fifth and Eighth Commandments, Luther's Small Catechism).

Health Education for All

God wants His Gospel shared with all people. He wants the benefits of His other blessings to be shared with all people as well, including those blessings that affect their physical well-being.

God's Word also teaches the following:

- God directs His people to pray and work for the good health and care of people everywhere. Jesus spent much time healing the sick and caring for those in need. Through His teaching, He urged His followers to do the same.

- "Speak up for those who cannot speak for themselves, for the rights of all who are destitute. Speak up and judge fairly; defend the rights of the poor and needy" (Proverbs 31:8–9 NIV). Working through the means of grace, God empowers those who belong to Him to provide food, clothing, shelter, and care for the unfortunate and to look to protect and enhance the lives of those unable to speak for themselves. This includes persons not yet born, those who are handicapped, and those not able to care for themselves. God's Spirit moves us to care for others unselfishly and unconditionally, and especially for those in need, even as Jesus sacrificially gave Himself for us and for all people.

- As God's Spirit empowers us, we practice good stewardship, caring for the resources God has given us. "Moreover, it is required of stewards that they be found trustworthy" (1 Corinthians 4:2). Good stewardship practices that affect the health of individuals may include

    taking care not to pollute air, land, and water;

    wisely using and managing natural resources and energy;

    recycling or reusing materials whenever possible;

    using the medicines and health care knowledge available for the good of all and the care of our own bodies.

Christian Education and Health Education

Christian educators believe that beneficial health education best occurs when people recognize God as the Creator and Sustainer of all life, when they trust Jesus Christ for forgiveness and new life, when they believe that He died to be the remedy for the malady of sin, and when they see caring for their own health and the health and safety of others as ways to bring honor and praise to the triune God—Father, Son, and Holy Spirit. Effective health instruction models the fruit of the Spirit (Galatians 5:22–23) by the power of the same Spirit, focuses on meeting the needs of the individual, and provides visually stimulating, accurate content from a Christian perspective, using a variety of instructional strategies.

It is the goal of the health volumes of the Concordia Curriculum Guide to equip and nurture the skills of teachers as they plan health education activities and policies for students and families that also proclaim God's great love for them, body and soul, given through the sacrificial life, death, and resurrection of His Son.

CHAPTER 3

National Health Standards: The Background for Health Education Programs in Christian Education

The American Association for Health Education (AAHE), in cooperation with the American Cancer Society, has developed the 2006 National Health Education Standards, PreK–12. These national standards provide a helpful organizing framework for health education standards as they are developed and implemented in the church's schools. They are presented in this chapter for your reference. The AAHE has given Concordia Publishing House permission to reprint the standards and to adapt them for use in Christian schools.

AAHE Standards for Health Education

Standard 1—Students will comprehend concepts related to health promotion and disease prevention to enhance health, as children of God through faith in Christ Jesus.

Standard 2—Students will analyze the influence of family, peers, culture, media, technology, and other factors on health behaviors as members of the body of Christ.

Standard 3—Students will demonstrate the ability to access valid information and products and services to enhance health as they are motivated through the means of grace to live their life for Him who lived, died, and rose again for them.

Standard 4—As they are empowered and guided by the Holy Spirit through God's Word, students will demonstrate the ability to use interpersonal communication skills to enhance health and avoid or reduce health risks.

Standard 5—In response to God's grace to them through Christ Jesus, students will demonstrate the ability to use decision-making skills to enhance health.

Standard 6—Students will demonstrate the ability to use goal-setting skills to enhance health, in loving service to our God and Savior.

Standard 7—Students will demonstrate the ability to practice health-enhancing behaviors, learning to avoid or reduce risks, as part of the new life they have been given to live by the Holy Spirit.

Standard 8—Together with their fellow believers, students will demonstrate the ability to advocate for personal, family, and community health.

These standards are cited from the prepublication document of National Health Education Standards, PreK–12. American Cancer Society. December 2005–April 2006. Reprinted with permission from the American Association for Health Education/AHPERD.

Consider the following questions as a faculty as you assess school-wide needs and evaluate and improve your health curriculum.

Discussion Questions

1. What insights do 1 Corinthians 6:19–20; 15:3; and 1 Timothy 4:4–5 provide to help children develop a healthy image of themselves and their bodies? What other Scripture passages may provide additional help to parents and children?

2. How do we as teachers help and equip students in the choices they make with respect to health and related behavioral issues? How do we work with others on these issues out of concern for them and love for our Savior? How do we express our love and concern?

3. What are some strategies that we might use to help parents work with their children to devel-

op a healthy, confident self-image, rooted in God and His love through Christ Jesus?

4. Which health-care professionals in our community might provide help to us and to our students and parents in promoting healthy behaviors and Christlike attitudes toward the human body and its functioning?

5. How might our health-care ministry in the school be part of a congregation-wide health-care ministry?

CHAPTER 4

Health Curriculum Standards for Students in Grade 6

The health education standards that are presented in this chapter are informed by the American Association for Health Education (AAHE) National Health Education Standards presented in the previous chapter and the health standards and performance expectations developed by the health education committees of the individual states. In order to offer a well-coordinated curriculum design, the health education objectives for each grade level are related to and connected with the standards provided at other grade levels. Teachers and schools are invited to use the CD that is included in the *Concordia Curriculum Guide: Health* at each grade level to modify the Concordia Health Education Standards for use in their own particular situation.

This chapter includes health standards that have been compiled from the individual state departments of education. They are organized grade by grade into the following seven areas:

1. Healthy Lifestyles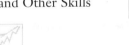

2. Health Information and Resources

3. Health Risks and Disease Prevention

4. Health Influencers

5. Health Goals and Decision Making

6. Health Communication and Other Skills

7. Health Advocacy

The Concordia standards have been systematized according to the following numerical designations to indicate grade level, category, and performance objective:

- The first digit indicates the grade level (e.g., the *2* in *2.5.1* designates that the performance expectation is for grade 2).
- The second digit indicates the standard number in health education being addressed (e.g., the *5* in *2.5.1* designates that the fifth health standard for grade 2 is being addressed).
- The third digit indicates the number of the specific performance expectation being addressed (e.g., the *1* in *2.5.1*, as found in the health standards of grade 2, relates to using accurate information when making health related decisions). The number of these expectations will vary from level to level.

The Concordia Health Education Standards for this grade level are stated below. Chapter 5 provides faith-integration activities organized according to each standard for this particular grade level. These activities provide many opportunities to teach aspects of the Christian faith in conjunction with each area of the health curriculum.

HEALTHY LIFESTYLES

6.1 **Sixth-grade students in Lutheran schools will understand concepts related to healthy lifestyles and the prevention of disease.**

6.1.1 Describe and explain the structure and function of the systems of the human body.

6.1.2 Identify responsible behaviors that help people maintain good health, and relate these behaviors to the prevention of injury, illness, disease, and premature death.

6.1.3 Explain the importance of assuming responsibility for their own personal health.

6.1.4 Explain how personal health habits, including daily vigorous exercise, influence the functioning of body systems.

6.1.5 Describe the relationships between a person and their surroundings and how one's surroundings influence physical, mental, social, and emotional health.

6.1.6 Explain ways to reduce risks related to common health problems of adolescents, and implement these ideas into their own lifestyle.

6.1.7 Describe how pathogens are related to the cause and prevention of disease.

6.1.8 Know and use key health and medical terms appropriately.

6.1.9 Know why some drugs are illegal, why they should not be used, and the consequences of their use.

6.1.10 Know the nutritional values of a variety of foods.

HEALTH INFORMATION AND RESOURCES

6.2 **Sixth-grade students in Lutheran schools will begin to develop the skills to access reliable sources of health information, understand the meaning of symbols on health products, and identify people who can answer health-related questions and provide health-related services.**

6.2.1 Develop and use guidelines to select health resources and use home, school, and community resources that provide reliable health information.

6.2.2 Analyze how media sources attempt to influence their choice of health information, products, and services.

6.2.3 Make comparison studies of the costs of basic health products.

6.2.4 Identify sources of health services in their community, and identify the roles of health care specialists in providing services.

HEALTH RISKS AND DISEASE PREVENTION

6.3   **Sixth-grade students in Lutheran schools will live in ways that enhance their own health and reduce or eliminate health risks.**

6.3.1   Demonstrate the ability to identify their own health needs and to understand their own responsibility for practicing good personal hygiene.

6.3.2   Compare and contrast safe and unsafe behaviors.

6.3.3   Demonstrate skills that enable them to positively deal with stress, grief, and anger.

6.3.4   Develop injury prevention and management skills to enhance personal and family health.

6.3.5   Demonstrate ways to recognize, avoid, and seek help in threatening situations.

6.3.6   Know and rehearse basic safety and health practices for personal and family health.

6.3.7   Develop the ability to analyze a personal health assessment to determine health needs and to develop strategies to improve and maintain personal health.

HEALTH INFLUENCERS

6.4   **Sixth-grade students in Lutheran schools will begin to understand that a variety of influences, including the media, the culture, and various technologies affect our thoughts, feelings, and perceptions about healthy behavior.**

6.4.1   Describe how their family, school, and peers influence their personal health behaviors.

6.4.2   Explore the roles culture, gender, and age differences have in personal health practices.

6.4.3   Describe how various media and technologies provide information and influence our attitudes about health practices.

6.4.4   Understand and accept that some people have special health needs.

HEALTH GOALS AND DECISION MAKING

6.5   **Sixth-grade students in Lutheran schools will set goals and use decision-making skills to enhance their own health and the health of others.**

6.5.1   Know how to identify and use appropriate sources of information when making health-related decisions.

6.5.2   Use a decision-making process to enhance their own health and solve health problems, individually and collaboratively.

6.5.3   Know how to set and make progress toward achieving a personal health and wellness goal.

6.5.4   Be able to predict how choices regarding reducing, reusing, and recycling have consequences for themselves and for others.

HEALTH COMMUNICATION AND OTHER SKILLS

6.6 **Sixth-grade students in Lutheran schools will develop interpersonal communication and other skills to better their own and others' health.**

6.6.1 Develop both verbal and nonverbal skills to communicate feelings, wants, and needs and to use nonviolent behaviors to resolve conflict.

6.6.2 Develop a variety of ways to communicate care, respect, and consideration for others.

6.6.3 Develop the characteristics needed to be a responsible friend and family member.

6.6.4 Use attentive listening skills to build healthy relationships.

6.6.5 Practice and be able to assertively use refusal and negotiation skills in potentially harmful situations.

6.6.6 Analyze causes of conflict among adolescents and develop the skill to use positive, nonviolent strategies to resolve conflict.

HEALTH ADVOCACY

6.7 **Sixth-grade students in Lutheran schools will develop the ability to advocate for healthy lifestyles for themselves, their family, and the community.**

6.7.1 Analyze the accuracy of health information, and use various methods to communicate reliable information and ideas about health matters.

6.7.2 Know ways to help and support others in making healthy choices.

6.7.3 Know about community agencies that support healthy families and provide activities that promote good health.

6.7.4 Demonstrate the ability to work cooperatively to achieve health goals for themselves, their families, and their community.

CHAPTER 5

Information and Activities for Integrating the Faith as Keyed to Grade 6 Standards

The health education standards included in this chapter have been compiled from the individual state departments of education and organized grade by grade into the following seven areas:

1. Healthy Lifestyles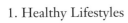

2. Health Information and Resources

3. Health Risks and Disease Prevention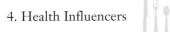

4. Health Influencers

5. Health Goals and Decision Making

6. Health Communication and Other Skills

7. Health Advocacy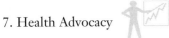

The standards have been systematized according to the following numerical designations to indicate grade level, category, and performance objective as described on the first page of chapter 4.

Performance expectations are numbered sequentially (e.g., the *4* in *7.1.4* is found in the grade 7 area, relating to *Healthy Lifestyles* and is the fourth item in that category). A complete list of health standards performance expectations for this grade level is provided in chapter 4.

On the pages of chapter 5, you will find an easy-to-reference two-column format for faith integration with the health standards. The left-hand column under the heading "Information by Topic" provides helpful teaching background information and insights relevant for integrating some aspect of the Christian faith. The number following the topic identifies the performance expectation to which the topic relates (see chapter 4). Beside each entry, in the right-hand column under the heading "Discussion Points/Activities," you will find ideas for student activities that nurture the Christian faith as students work to achieve the related health standard.

Be sure to consult the index at the end of this volume for a complete listing of topics and where they may be found.

HEALTHY LIFESTYLES

6.1   **Sixth-grade students in Lutheran schools will understand concepts related to healthy lifestyles and the prevention of disease.**

Systems of the Human Body (Skeletal, Muscular, Respiratory)

Much of what goes on beneath a person's skin takes place by God's gracious design and without any specific direction or thought on the part of the owner. It is only when something goes wrong that a person's attention is drawn to the muscle or tissue inside his or her body. How often does that same description apply to your relationship with Jesus? Our hearts beat, our lungs breathe, and our stomachs digest. When pain comes to visit, many often want to be rid of it as soon as possible, not realizing it is truly a great gift. Jesus Christ chose to live within the confines of a human body, indicating how much He values this earthly flesh and would have us do the same. Our pain is a reminder of the suffering, pain, and death He took on Himself so that we might be saved from sin's eternal pain. Through His suffering, we have everlasting life with Him. He took the pain of our sin on Himself and freed us to live with and for Him each day. Through our healing, He is honored. (6.1.1)

• Research the five senses, summarize their tasks, and choose an art medium to design a sculpture, montage, or collage depicting the function of each sense. How does one sense carry on the work of another should something happen to it? Share your artwork with your class, and discuss the blessings God provides to us through these senses. If you had to give up one of your senses, which would it be? Explain your choice.
• The human skeletal system is made up of 206 bones and many joints and hinges. One of its most important components is the opposable thumb. Tell your partner what you think are the two main functions of the skeleton. How is the skeleton like the rules of a game? Compare and contrast the work of the skeletal system with the uses of God's Law as spelled out in Luther's explanations to the Ten Commandments. Without structure (or laws), there would be pandemonium and chaos. How does God's Law provide structure for human life?

Behaviors, Responsible

Paul's words in 1 Corinthians 6:19–20 remind us that we do not have the right to do anything we want to or with our bodies, for in reality our body does not belong to us. God created us and Jesus Christ redeemed us from the bondage of sin and death. It has been said that we are twice bought. Our bodies are temples of the Holy Spirit. Talk about pressure! I'm anxious over the fact that someone may accidentally forget to use a coaster and cause a water stain on my new furniture. Sure, the table cost me a fair amount of money, but nothing like the cost Jesus paid on my behalf. Because of His love for me, I take care to honor my body by watching what I put into it, by treating it with the love Jesus has shown me, and by working with others to glorify God in all I do. (6.1.2)

• Choose a sport that requires participants to wear protective gear of one kind or another. Identify the vulnerable body parts in this sport, and describe the gear worn to protect them. Our faith is also vulnerable to attack from Satan, the father of lies. What protective gear has God given you to help defend against Satan's wily ways (Ephesians 6:10–18)?
• Do research online or perhaps at your local hospital's emergency center to find information regarding typical seasonal accidents. Make a chart showing your findings. Use pictures or words to describe the activity and charts or graphs to show the statistics relating to injuries, then identify the safe behavior(s) or precaution(s) that may have prevented the injury. Discuss the relationship of the behavior to a commandment that God gave. What is one reason for obeying the commandments (1 John 4:19)?

Health, Responsibility for

In his explanation to the First Article, Martin Luther writes an extensive list of how God created us, how He richly and daily provides for us, and how He defends us. There is nothing we need to do or be in order for our heavenly Father to act in such a loving and caring manner. We cannot earn God's favor, we don't deserve it, and we don't have to remind Him that we are down here waiting. More likely we go on our ways without too much thought about all that is being done on our behalf. This reminds me of the manner in which hearts keep beating, lungs breathing, and stomachs digesting—all without any thought or effort on our part. Luther goes on to remind us why God acts and what response we should have: "All this He does only out of fatherly, divine goodness and mercy, without any merit or worthiness in me. For all this it is my duty to thank and praise, serve and obey Him" (From *Luther's Small Catechism with Explanation*, © 1986, 1991, 2005 CPH, p. 16). Everything we need is provided; all that is required of us is to receive what is given. Understanding the enormity of the gift, we can't help but follow through with this "duty." (6.1.3)

• Interview your parents or guardians about the things they needed to do for you during the early years of your life, such as until you were five. As you grew, what changes were required to provide for your nutritional needs, safe space (baby proofing), toilet training, and developing good hygiene habits? Using pictures from magazines, grocery-store ads, catalogs, and perhaps pictures from your early childhood, design a collage that portrays the ways your parents assumed responsibility for your health and care. Place the words of Isaiah 38:16, 19 on your collage: "O Lord . . . the father makes known to the children Your faithfulness."

• As a sixth grader, you no longer require the same level of supervision and care you once did. At the same time, you are not yet able to handle making all your own decisions. What level of responsibility have you assumed for your own health? Take a personal inventory of things you do or do not do that impact your health. Write a list of at least three responsibilities you maintain and three responsibilities you often leave undone. How is assessing your responsibility for your own health similar to what John says about assessing our behavior in 1 John 1:8–10?

Health Habits

In Jesus' day, nearly all the activities of daily living provided a natural physical fitness component. A person's body systems benefited by this level of activity. Traveling was done on foot. Carpenters would have done everything by hand, including cutting the tree, hauling it to the shop, and doing all the preparation to make the wood right for the project at hand. Women walked long distances to the wells for water and carried heavy jars on the return trip. Meal preparation involved physical labor, and faithful Jews practiced very strict dietary laws. Contemporary studies suggest the health benefits of physical exercise and following these dietary laws. Yet Paul recognized that his salvation was not due to his efforts but to God's grace alone in Christ Jesus (Ephesians 2:8–9). As you encourage students to participate in vigorous activity regularly, share with them the joy of God's gifts to them in Christ Jesus. (6.1.4)

• What is the current definition of a physically fit body? To develop a definition, consult the Web site Fitness Fundamentals (www.hoptechno.com/book11.htm), created by the President's Council on Physical Fitness and Sports. Describe the four or five basic components of physical fitness, identify the organ systems involved, and demonstrate exercises that can help test or improve physical fitness. What are some activities that will increase your spiritual fitness (Acts 2:42–47)?

• Simple walking is a great fitness activity. The Web site for Kids Walk-to-School, www.cdc.gov/nccdphph/dnpa/kidswalk/index.htm, will help you start an organized walking program in your school. If your school draws from a wide area, perhaps you should concentrate on a Kids Walk-to-VBS in your church's neighborhood. Walking together can remind you of the people who walked from place to place, following Jesus and listening to Him teach.

Influences on Health (Physical, Mental, Social, Emotional)

When the Pharisees once tried to trick Jesus with questions, they asked which commandment was the greatest (Matthew 22:34–40; Mark 12:28–34). Jesus gave a two-pronged response. He first quoted the Shema from Deuteronomy 6:4, and added "a second is like it: You shall love your neighbor as yourself" (Matthew 22:39). In Hebrew parlance, Jesus' language choice said that the two were actually equal in importance. Loving God with all your being is a vertical direction, while loving your neighbor as yourself is horizontal in nature. Notice the cross-style living this implies. We cannot love our neighbor without first knowing God's love. Jesus showed us by word and deed how to do both. Psalm 1 is a beautiful illustration of the life of one who obeys God and chooses friends carefully. Our relationships can influence us to live in the joy of Jesus or drive us to follow Satan's temptations. In His Word, God provides sure guidance for our lives and the clear Gospel of forgiveness and love offered to all people in His Son. Help your students develop close relationships with people who treasure God's Word and use it faithfully. (6.1.5)

• Psalm 1 describes life with God as a tree planted by streams of water. Some family trees may look like actual trees as names are added to the various branches. Consider the friends and family who support and encourage you in your walk with Jesus, those people who hold you accountable to walk the talk. Design an image of a family tree close to a stream. Its branches and leaves should be strong and beautiful. Add the names or other representations of the people on your spiritual family tree, the ones who nurture you in faith. A tree's root system is as broad as its visible canopy, and its job is to provide sturdiness, gather water to send up the trunk, and feed the branches and tips that are far out. What or who makes up the root system of your tree? Label the roots of your tree as you wish. Thank God for all parts of your faith family tree that help keep you spiritually safe.

• What or who serve as negative influences, those who do not honor and encourage your choices to follow God's will and live in Jesus' joy? In which of the areas mentioned in the standard above do you feel the most vulnerable? How can members of your class or those in your spiritual family tree help you stand firm in faith? In a letter, tell your classmates how they can encourage and support you in your spiritual growth.

Health Problems

Over many years, science has worked diligently to create and refine vaccines and other medicines to help human beings fight the various diseases that plagued the generations before us. As much as technology would like to take the credit, we know that it is God who gave these men and women the minds and the skills, the creative thinking, and the ability to follow through one hypothesis after another to develop these vaccines and medications. As God continues to guide and bless the work done to protect the health of children, we thank Him for the cure for the sin that infects all of us that He has provided in His Son. (6.1.6)

• On the Internet, visit www.kidshealth.org/kid/, and you will find a plethora of articles and interesting information about you and your body. Once you have found the home page, click on "Everyday Illnesses and Injuries." Choose one, and write a brief report about an illness or injury that affects teens. Also provide information about the prevention and treatment of this disease or injury. How did Jesus deal with the sting of injury and death (1 Corinthians 15:54–57)?

• "Cover your mouth." "Wash your hands!" "Keep your hands away from your face!" These and other common phrases are often heard during the cold and flu season. Using the same site listed above, search for the section on "Chilling Out with Colds." Team with a partner to put together a puppet show appropriate for younger children in which you teach them proper ways to prevent catching or spreading a cold. With the teacher, arrange an appropriate time to share your play. Remind the students how God has taken away the ache and pain of sin through the suffering, death, and resurrection of Jesus and the cleansing waters of our Baptism.

Pathogens

A pathogen or infectious agent is a biological agent that causes disease or illness to its host. The word *pathogen* comes from the Greek and means "birth of pain." When God created humankind, He included a very efficient immune system to deal with pathogens making their way into our bodies. Secondary to this line of defense is a group of helpful bacteria that join forces with our immune system to fight off diseases. A person who has a compromised or weakened disease-fighting team will be more vulnerable to opportunistic infections. There are times in our spiritual lives when we are extremely vulnerable to Satan and his infections. Doubt, worry, too many problems at one time—any or all of these can fool us into forgetting that God is always on our side, wanting the best and most bountiful of blessings for each of His children. It's at times such as these that God's Word, such as His Word in Romans 8:31–39, sustains us with the healing fragrances provided by God through His Son (2 Corinthians 2:14–16). (6.1.7)

• We live in an environment where both helpful and harmful pathogens exist side by side. If we are prescribed an antibiotic for one illness, it may well kill some of the helpful germs living in our bodies and make it possible for other infections to take hold. What are some ways in which your body can become vulnerable to pathogens? Name two pathogens that especially afflict people of your age, describe the symptoms of the disease, and identify two treatments that might be used to fight the disease. For help consult "The Bad Bug Book" at www.cfsan.fda.gov/~mow/intro.html. Name several spiritual pathogens that threaten our faith in Jesus. What medicines does God prescribe for us (1 Peter 1:24–25)?

• What can you do to ensure that the foods you serve or eat are safe? Study this food-safety Web site at www.extension.iastate.edu/foodsafety/lesson/?CFID=3688312&CFTOKEN=93150942. Then make a poster that features several rules for food safety. What advice does God give us regarding faith safety? Consult these Scripture passages: Romans 16:17–18; Ephesians 4:1–6; 6:10–18; Colossians 3:1–4; and 2 Timothy 3:14–17. Create a companion poster to the food-safety poster that features several rules for faith safety. Include creative titles on your posters. Display your posters together.

Terms (Health, Medical)

As you teach to this standard, help students also to acquire the key grace and mercy terms of the Gospel of Jesus Christ, key terms regarding worship, and a rich vocabulary for prayer. Check yourself periodically to make certain you are not assuming your students understand this key vocabulary. Through His teaching and His sacrificial death and resurrection to life, Jesus, the master teacher, made certain His audience knew by faith

• Because of the sin of Adam and Eve, we no longer live in a Garden of Eden environment. Perfection has been replaced by the consequences of sin, and illness is one of them. To become familiar with some pathogens, make a three-column chart with the words *Pathogen*, *Examples*, and *Typical Effects* across the top. In the first column headed "Pathogen," write, "Bacteria, Viruses, Protozoa, Fungi, and Parasites." For each of these

that He was the Lamb of God sent to save all people from their sins. (6.1.8)

pathogens, do research and give two examples and the typical effects experienced from each one. On your chart, place God's promise to "wipe away every tear" from those washed in the blood of the Lamb (Revelation 7:14–17).

• Together with your classmates, prepare reports about each of the following topics: anorexia, bulimia, cystic fibrosis, hemophilia, sickle cell anemia, and Tay-Sachs disease. In each report, include information about groups that support research and treatment for that health problem. Gather the reports into a Big Book of Health. Add to the collection with other health reports made during the year. Prepare short quizzes about each report for classmates to take. For a preface for your collection, write a prayer asking God to bless the research being done to treat various diseases and to bring comfort and help to those who suffer. Explore the ways your collection might be made available to others using technology.

Drugs (Illegal Use of, Consequences)

Today's teens are pulled and pushed in every direction to "get this," "wear that," and "try this." Their world is one where drugs are readily available, sexual innuendo is often used in advertising and humor, and security-system checkpoints at the school's entrance hope to keep the surroundings safe. The temptation to go along with the crowd is strong. The story of Jesus' temptation (Matthew 4:1–11) is an excellent lesson for anyone facing such pressure. Your students will have learned that Jesus was also a teen and had to deal with many of the same issues they do, just under different circumstances. As you discuss each of the three temptations Satan put before Jesus, brainstorm what situation might be its counterpart in your students' world. Note how Jesus responded, and develop some appropriate behaviors for them to model as they respond to temptation. Remind your class that not only can Jesus identify with them, but He also provides the power and desire to equip them to conquer these temptations with His Word. (6.1.9)

• Using what you learned about the temptation of Jesus in the wilderness, draw a six-panel cartoon-style story showing a student being tempted to try an illegal substance. What temptation is put before him or her? What thought process goes on in his or her head? What responses, similar to Jesus' responses, may be given to indicate he or she is not interested? If you prefer, choose a partner and write this situation as a role play and perform it for your class.

• Conduct a computer search to discover the relationship between drinking and automobile accidents involving teens. Show your results on a chart or graph. One source of information is www.onlinelawyersource.com/personal_injury/car/teen.html. Write a safe driving pledge for teens. See this Web site for ideas: www.fbfs.com/fbfs/Rhythmyx/content/resources/teen_pledge.pdf. What Bible verse do you think would be a good companion verse for such a driving pledge?

Foods, Nutritional Value of

The Bible makes many references to food. In the Old Testament, the dietary laws regarding clean and unclean animals were one of God's ways to keep His children healthy. In the New Testament, Jesus celebrated feasts and other occasions with food, fed multitudes of people with small amounts of food, and called Himself the bread of life (John 6:35). In Holy Communion, we eat and drink bread and wine and also receive Jesus' body and blood; this meal is a foretaste of the feast to come. While on earth, we may struggle to keep a balanced diet of nutritious foods, not always understanding good fat versus bad fat. In Jesus' body and blood, given for us and for our salvation, there can be no doubt! It is the bread of life—pure love, pure forgiveness, and pure strength to go on. May it be so for you also! (6.1.10)

• Visit www.nal.usda.gov/fnic/Fpyr/pyramid.html for information about the Food Guide Pyramid. Click on the new section for kids to learn even more about how to evaluate the foods you eat. Choose a favorite family meal, and measure it against these guidelines. What changes can you make in this meal so that it is healthier for everyone in your family? Help prepare this meal. Make a centerpiece for your table in which you thank God for the food He provides. Use one of these verses or another one of your choosing as part of your centerpiece: Psalm 104:27–28; 111:4–5; 136:25.

• Make a poster advertising a nutritional food, such as broccoli. Create a cartoon character to advertise the nutritional qualities of the food. Entitle your poster "God's Power Food." Consult these Web sites for help: www.nutritiondata.com/ or www.ars.usda.gov/main/site_main.htm?mode code=12354500.

HEALTH INFORMATION AND RESOURCES

INFORMATION BY TOPIC

DISCUSSION POINTS/ACTIVITIES

6.2   Sixth-grade students in Lutheran schools will begin to develop the skills to access reliable sources of health information, understand the meaning of symbols on health products, and identify people who can answer health-related questions and provide health-related services.

Health Resources

As important as guidelines are for selecting reliable health resources, it is even more important that we depend on reliable guidelines when we select resources that are to nurture our spiritual health. Our gracious God has written the Law first on our hearts and then on the two tablets of stone given to Moses (the Ten Commandments). Knowing that no one could keep His Law perfectly, God sent Jesus, His Word made flesh, to be the perfect guideline—an exemplar if you wish—who showed us in words and actions what it means to live in love. He kept the Law perfectly for us. He died to suffer our penalty for not keeping God's Law and rose from the dead to proclaim victory over sin and Satan. Now, He gives us His resurrection power to lead lives that honor Him. Indeed, we love because He first loved us (1 John 4:19). The Bible is our primary resource from which we learn about God's love for us in Jesus Christ and receive His power to respond to that love with love toward others (Psalm 119:105; 1 Thessalonians 2:13). (6.2.1)

• Making sure that information is reliable and true is an important part of life. Read about the Queen of Sheba's evaluation of Solomon in 1 Kings 10:1–10. About what did she ask? How did she determine if the things she had heard were true? We need to carefully evaluate health information also. Medline Plus (www.nlm.nih.gov/medlineplus/evaluatinghealthinformation.html), a service of the National Library of Medicine, provides articles to help people evaluate the reliability of health materials. Read several of these articles, and make a list of the features of an article that would indicate whether or not the health information in the article is reliable. Discuss your list with your classmates and teacher.

• To provide guidance for those who wish to give blood for use in the community, develop brochures based on information provided by the American Red Cross and other agencies that collect blood. There is another type of blood already given for you that you can read about in the following Bible references: Romans 5:6–11; Ephesians 1:7–10; 1 Peter 1:18–19; 1 John 1:7; and Revelation 1:4–6. Look up three of the five Scripture references, and include in your brochure a brief paragraph sharing what you learned about this blood and its benefits for you and others in your community. How do you know that the information you receive from the Red Cross materials is reliable? How do you know that the information you receive about Jesus' blood from Scripture is reliable (2 Timothy 3:14–17)?

• Make a health-information list for the people living in your home. Include in this list any chronic illnesses, allergies, special needs, and types of medication each person is using. On a separate sheet, list emergency telephone numbers and the names and phone numbers of your primary-care doctors. Finally, place this information in a portfolio and keep it by the telephone. You could also make a spiritual-health information list. Include a reminder to pray (Jesus' 911 emergency number), special Bible verses that are meaningful to you, and the names and telephone numbers of people you know you can call for help.

Media (Health Information)

Remember the parable of the two men? One built his house on rock, the other on sand (Matthew 7:24–27). When the rains, the floods, and the wind came crashing down upon the house on the rock, it stood solid because its foundation was strong. The house with the foundation of sand suffered the same climatic calamities and could not withstand them. It tumbled down. In this parable, Jesus teaches that wise folks build their houses of faith and trust on His foundation, His truth. Jesus Christ is the foundation on which the Christian Church is built (1 Corinthians 3:11); instruction about that foundation is found in God's Word, the writings and teachings of the apostles and prophets (Ephesians 2:19–20). When we hear, learn, and obey God's Word, the Holy Spirit secures us in the faith and frees us from the fear of collapsing into the world's way rather than God's way. No matter how much Satan, sin, and self call to us to go that way or give in on this small point of contention, our foundation is sure and we can more easily say, "Thanks, but no thanks!" (6.2.2)

• Talk with your grandparent or a person at least two generations older than you about the remedies they use to soothe a sore throat, an earache, an itchy case of mosquito bites, or some other ailment. How did they learn of this remedy? Were these remedies purchased at the pharmacy or learned from their parents and grandparents? Describe what you learned. Is the success of a product a good advertising tool? What long-lasting remedy for sin do Christians share with others (Ephesians 5:25–27)?

• As you watch television, notice that commercials are not the only techniques used to sway people to purchase a product. Product placement in the show itself is a very subtle way to encourage people to buy certain items; watch for the brand of soda on the table or the sign on the wall. Ask your classmates to list the products they see in the TV shows they watch. Compile a list of all of these products. What products do Christians place near people to expose people to the message of the Gospel? What Christian products are in your home that may expose visitors to Jesus Christ, our Savior? Name some items, and discuss how these items may help bring the Gospel to others. What products might you make more visible in your home to tell others about Jesus?

Costs (Health Product Comparisons)

Old movies depict snake-oil salesman moving from town to town trying to sell their special elixir, guaranteeing that it will cure just about any ailment one might have. Often the elixir was nothing more than alcohol. People paid a high price and received no cure. The Bible warns about false prophets who claim they have special knowledge or abilities to help people but have no cure. Jesus

• What features would you look for in a Band-Aid or a cough drop? Make a list of the features you feel are important in the health product you are researching. Make an appointment at a local pharmacy to interview one of the staff people about the features of various Band-Aids or another health product you use. Ask questions about the various features and costs of the products, record

went from village to village teaching and healing. He charged no one for His services. Following the resurrection, the timid disciples were turned into evangelists who couldn't help but share the great Good News of Jesus Christ, the risen Lord and Savior. No snake oil here; no asking for any amount of money. Jesus' resurrection is powerful proof that God's grace and forgiveness is a real cure for sin. The Gospel of Jesus Christ is given as a free gift. It cannot be bought; it can only be received. It is all grace. A person who knows the Gospel freely shares what was freely given. As students compare costs of health care, help them keep in mind that the greatest health care of all time, the cure of our sin sickness, cost the greatest sum imaginable, so high that only one man, a God-man, could pay the price. And He did—once and for all! Jesus gave His life for our salvation (2 Corinthians 5:14–15), and we receive it as a gift. (6.2.3)

the answers you receive, and make a comparison chart showing the features of the health products you study. Share your findings with your class. Be certain to write a thank you note to the person who gave you some of his or her time for the interview. How is this process similar to the activity the apostle John advised Christians to engage in whenever they were invited to trust in a savior other than Jesus (1 John 4:1–3)?

• People like to get a suntan, but they also use sun block or sunscreen to prevent injury to their skin. What benefits to people does exposure to the sun bring? Use the Internet or visit a pharmacy to research and compare the ingredients and the cost of various types of sun block. Be sure to compare the cost per ounce. Write a radio commercial to advertise your recommendation as the best sun block for your classmates to use; present your ad to your class. Reflect on Psalm 84:11. Why does the psalmist describe God as being both a sun and a shield, perhaps from the sun?

Health Services, Community Specialists

Jesus, the Great Physician, was both a general practitioner and a specialist who cared deeply about the people who crowded around Him so that they might hear His voice and perhaps be healed by His hand. As a healer, Jesus looked not only at the physical body of the individual before Him but also paid close attention to the spiritual healing that was needed. Recall the story (Mark 2:1–12) of the man whose four friends let him down through the roof to be healed by Jesus. Jesus was first concerned that the man receive forgiveness of sins. That was His specialty. He healed the man of his physical ills to show that He also had the "authority on earth to forgive sins" (Mark 2:10). May the Lord's Spirit bless you as you engage in your specialty—nurturing faith in our Savior, Jesus. (6.2.4)

• One of the quickest ways to identify sources of health care in your community would be to look in the Yellow Pages under "Physicians." Search for the names of four different specialists in your area. On separate pages of a small booklet, write their names, specialties, and other information about their medical practice. On each page, place a footnote defining any unfamiliar terms that name the physician's specialty. On the last page of the booklet, write a description of Jesus' specialty. He is our Great Physician.

• Nurses, radiologists—the people who read x-rays—physical and occupational therapists, psychiatrists, psychologists, therapists, and counselors all help people in different ways. Find a prayer that your church uses to pray for health-care professionals. Pray it with your class during your class devotions.

HEALTH RISKS AND DISEASE PREVENTION

6.3   **Sixth-grade students in Lutheran schools will live in ways that enhance their own health and reduce or eliminate health risks.**

Personal Health and Hygiene

Jesus warned His followers about seeing a speck in their brother's eye but not noticing the log in their own eye (Matthew 7:3). He also warned about the folly of offering to remove the defects in others that we don't see in ourselves. While these verses are pointed most directly at judging others, they also remind us to take care of our own health-care needs as we teach others about health. The American Medical Association provides guidelines concerning what tests adults should have at various ages. For one such listing, see www.healthgoods. com/education/health_information/Personal_Health/personal_checkup.htm. These recommendations take into consideration family history, ethnicity, and one's own health history. It is so much easier to encourage a spouse, sibling, or parent to get that test taken care of than to have your own regular checkups. Ecclesiastes tells us two are better than one for a variety of reasons (Ecclesiastes 4:9–12). Be a good role model for your students as you teach to this standard. Buddy up with a friend or family member, and keep current on your own health-care needs. (6.3.1)

• By now you have learned quite a bit about what you need to do to stay healthy. Your parents make sure you get to doctor visits for shots and check-ups, the dentist to keep your teeth healthy, and perhaps the orthodontist if you need braces. At each place, you have been taught how to practice good hygiene in order to be as healthy as possible. Make a poster encouraging your classmates to get regular checkups to enable them to care for the bodies God has given them.

• Your church youth group is going on an overnight retreat. The facility will take care of your meals and snacks and provide mattresses and bunk beds for sleeping. Make a list of the personal health-care items you will need to put in your backpack or gym bag for this event. Would you consider your Bible and devotional materials personal health-care items?

Behaviors, Safe and Unsafe

If your staff shares playground duty, it is quite likely you look over a crowd of people and find yourself on the lookout for safe and unsafe behaviors. Read Psalm 91. What a comfort it is to know that we are always in the safety of our Father's hand, even when we have made a stupid move because our mind was not focused on the task at hand. Jesus was consoled by this psalm. It was also used by Satan to tempt our Lord while He fasted in the wilderness. Be open to recognizing, even in your busiest times, the moments when God has kept you safe. Teach your students to see God's caring hand in the work of medical, police, and fire-fighting personnel. (6.3.2)

• Review Psalm 139, and recall how God made us in just the right way so that we could best serve Him as we serve others. Learn and sing the Michael Joncas song called "On Eagle's Wings" (*LSB* 727). Think about the words describing how God holds us safely in the palm of His hand.

• Riding in cars is a great way to get from one place to another. Using seatbelts is one way to increase travel safety. Some may feel seatbelts are too restrictive or too much hassle for a short trip. In some states, tickets are issued if passengers are not wearing proper restraints. Babies and little children have unique needs for car travel safety. Find out what the rules regarding seatbelt use are in your state. Find some statistics about accidents and what impact seatbelt wearing and child protective positioning had in the welfare of those involved. Make an effort to talk with someone whose life was saved because seatbelts were used. Investigate several Bible passages that encourage people to take good care of their bodies. Report your findings in a PowerPoint presentation if that technology is available; otherwise use posters, graphs, and pictures to share what you learned.

Skills to Deal with (Stress, Grief, Anger)

How did our Savior deal with stress? Many days He was busy with teaching, healing the sick, and traveling from one place to another. When He felt stressed, He withdrew to a place where He could pray (Luke 5:15–16). To the strategies for dealing with stress suggested for your students at the Kids Health Web site (www.kidshealth.org/kid/feeling/), add prayer. The Lord invites you to pray and to lay all your cares on Him because He cares for you (Zechariah 10:3; 1 Peter 5:7). Some useful ideas for helping students develop the skills to manage anger in God-pleasing ways are available in Unit 5 of *Getting Along: Peaceful Problem Solving Skills for the Christian Classroom* (St. Louis, Concordia Publishing House, 1996). (6.3.3)

• Make a list of things that cause you stress. Did you include any useful stress? Some stress is useful. Consider a violin or guitar string. If no stress is put upon it, it will be limp and unable to make any sound at all. Tighten the peg to just the right tension and a perfectly-pitched tone can be produced! Distress is negative stress and eustress is positive. Read about stress at www.kidshealth.org. Click on "Kids," then choose "Dealing with Feelings" from the menu, and then scroll down until you reach "My Emotions and Behaviors." From this section, read several articles about stress. List things you can do to relieve stress. Read 1 Peter 5:7, and add Peter's suggestion for dealing with stress to your list. Make a bookmark that has your ideas for dealing with stress on it.

• Plan ahead. In Minnesota, where the summer brings thunderstorms and the winter delivers snow and cold weather, many people pack a storm kit ahead of time so they are prepared to face emergencies. Items included in a storm kit are a flashlight, battery-operated radio, water, food, and blanket. Plan an emotional storm kit (ESK) for yourself so that you are prepared to handle stress, anger, and grief ahead of time and know exactly where to go for help. Brainstorm some of the things you might include in your ESK. You might include songs and hymns that encourage you, Bible verses that speak of God's love and comfort, names of people you know who will stand by you—even in the middle of the night (see Mark 2). Take this emotional storm kit home to your family and discuss handling stress, anger, and grief in ways that help everyone and bring honor and praise to God for His love shown to us in Jesus.

Injury Prevention and Family Health

The hymn "With the Lord Begin Your Task" (*LSB* 869, *LW* 483) contains fitting devotional thoughts related to this standard, whether applied to physical or spiritual health. Placing each day into Jesus' hands is not a magic potion against injury or harm. Rather, the hymn reminds us that the Lord Jesus is watching over and keeping us and all for whom we care safe from harm and the tempter's might. He will never be taken by surprise as He cares for us because He has already put into place all that is needed for the day's journey. Wherever the day leads, we are never alone because Jesus is always by our side. He gave His life for us. His management skills are beyond reproach, so approach each day confidently. His blessings will abound no matter what! (6.3.4)

• Create a home safety checklist. There are a number of home safety check sites on the Internet that may serve as a model. The checklist at www.umm.edu/non_trauma/check.htm is one good reference. Tour your house with pencil, checklist, and clipboard (You may wear a hard hat if you would like!) to make a home safety check. Be on the lookout for trouble spots—places or things that could cause accidents or injuries. Report your findings and suggestions for improvements to your family. Make a safe home certificate to display in your home. On it include this passage from Scripture: "Whoever trusts in the Lord is safe" (Proverbs 29:25).
• Does your family have a plan for a fire emergency? Do you conduct practice fire drills? If not, plan an agenda for a family meeting. Seek information about home fire escape planning from your local fire department and from www.usfa. fema.gov/safety/escape/. Present an escape plan to evacuate your home. Include escape routes and a place outside your home for members of your family to meet in an emergency. Encourage your family to practice your escape plans. Include on your meeting agenda a prayer asking God to keep your family safe from harm and danger.

Seeking Help in Threatening Situations

Throughout Jesus' ministry, He had to support and encourage disciples who were fearful and scared. The storms that were so scary to them must have been serious, considering that a number of the men were fishermen by trade and practically lived on the water. Because we know Jesus' full story from cradle to cross to crown, it is hard for us to understand how these twelve men could be so fearful in the midst of a storm when Jesus was right in the boat with them! And He was sleeping nonetheless! Keep in mind that they were still living each event in real time without knowing the outcome. My guess is that there are a many of us educators who would respond in the same manner. In our day, many potential weather dangers can be foreseen and response plans made. During the

• Weather situations and storms will differ, depending on where you live and the season of the year. Tornados, thunderstorms, blizzards, hurricanes—each one calls for a different type of preparation and protection. Arrange for a meteorologist from your local television station to visit your school and talk about causes and consequences of seasonal weather activity. Invite a firefighter or paramedic to speak about safety precautions and readiness plans. In your class prayer time or your own personal devotions, thank God for the knowledge and skills of these people as well as their willingness to work in risky situations.
• Design a book or write a skit to help younger children know how to be safe and how to get help when needed. The Lowell, Massachusetts, Police

2005–2006 school year, however, people were overwhelmed by extreme weather conditions. The wonder of nature morphed into a power so great that entire cities were demolished. It is important as you teach to this standard that students are reminded that, whatever the situation, "Jesus is in their boat," helping, protecting, and guiding. Balance is key. Help children recognize and avoid dangerous situations without engendering in them a paralyzing fear of what might happen. Assure your students with God's promises. "Fear not, for I am with you," God says. "I will help you, I will uphold you with My righteous right hand" (Isaiah 41:10). (6.3.5)

Department has provided a useful summary of suggestions for parents at www.lowellpolice.com/crime_safety/safety_tips/child_safety.htm. Use these ideas for your book or skit. Remember to include the idea that God provides many people who are trained and available to help us when we need it.

Health and Safety Practices

The Good Samaritan (Luke 10:25–37) is an example of a person making use of basic health practices in order to help someone else. To the Jews, a good Samaritan was an oxymoron; they were certainly not the people one would expect to stop and offer medical help! The Samaritan did what he could to help the man and went beyond the basics by putting the man up in an inn and paying for whatever care he needed. His loving action is an example for us to follow today. Encourage your children to learn safe ways to help those in need. Obtain certification in Red Cross Basic First Aid. Remind your students also that Jesus is the Good Samaritan for us. He has helped us in our most dire need. He paid the price for our forgiveness on the cross with His own life. (6.3.6)

• Work with your school nurse or other medical professional to learn the basics of providing first aid to someone in need. One summary of these basics is available from the National Ag Safety Database (www.cdc.gov/nasd/docs/d000101-d000200/d000105/d000105.html). Assemble a first aid kit for your classroom or examine the kit your teacher has for your room. Use the National Ag Safety Database list to help complete this project. What items need to be included? Which items should be changed periodically? Identify the situations in which each item would be helpful. Demonstrate or discuss the proper use of each item. Compare preparing to deal with an emergency to preparing for Jesus' appearance on the last day (1 Peter 1:13).

• Ask each of your classmates to research and report on how some of the following wounds should be treated: animal bites, burns, cuts, eye injuries, frostbite, nosebleeds, sprains, and sunburn. A useful resource is the HealthWorld Online Web site at www.healthy.net/scr/MainLinks.asp?Id=170. As you consider how to care for these various injuries, read and meditate on the apostle Peter's thought that Jesus bound up our wounds by being wounded Himself (1 Peter 2:21–24). "By His wounds you have been healed" (1 Peter 2:24).

Assessment, Health

This is the perfect standard to use for your own personal insight and growth. In each instance where the word *personal* is used, exchange it for the word *spiritual*. At times we get so caught up in our physical fitness that we forget about the spiritual state of our health. Decide on several markers that would indicate the state of your spiritual health and place them into a pyramid or another shape that might hold more symbolism for you. Examine these passages in Matthew to see how Jesus nurtured the spiritual health of His disciples: Matthew 5:1–2, 13–16; 6:33; 12:1–8; 13:18–23; 16:13–19; 18:21–22; 19:13–15; 28:9. Decide where you fall within this assessment, and then work with a partner to set up a covenant that supports activities in which your spiritual health will be nurtured and that are specific, measurable, and reasonable. As the Holy Spirit strengthens your relationship with Jesus through His Word and Sacraments, the fruit by which you are known will become more enticing and recognizable. Blessings on this journey! (6.3.7)

• Use the cool MyPyramid Tracker at mypyramid tracker.gov/ to assess your own food intake and physical activity. Team with a partner to create your own profiles, and encourage each other to eat healthily and exercise sufficiently to maintain optimum physical condition for yourselves. Working together will enable you to be more successful because of the encouragement, accountability, and fun you'll have creating new ways to be and eat healthy. Working together is an idea referred to in Ecclesiastes 4:9–12. Why is having at least one partner easier than trying to do a challenging thing on your own? Your team can also pray for one another and ask for protection from Satan, who will try to get you off track; ask Jesus to give you the courage and motivation you will need to maintain a healthy lifestyle.

• Use the Healthy Eating Calculator at www.kids nutrition.org/HealthyEating_calculator.htm to plan meals for a day based on the recommendations of the calculator. If you increased your physical activity, what changes could you make in your meals? Remember, your body is God's temple, and you want to treat it well (1 Corinthians 6:19–20).

HEALTH INFLUENCERS

INFORMATION BY TOPIC   DISCUSSION POINTS/ACTIVITIES

6.4   Sixth-grade students in Lutheran schools will begin to understand that a variety of influences, including the media, the culture, and various technologies, influence our thoughts, feelings, and perceptions about healthy behavior.

Influences, Health Behavior

In our humanness, we are all easily influenced, tempted, and even coerced into doing things we had planned not to do. Paul, who had this same concern, wrote, "I do not understand my own actions. For I do not do what I want, but I do the very thing I hate" (Romans 7:15). Satan has a way of making unhealthy activities, whether physical or spiritual, attractive. Even if I were alone on a desert island, temptations would assail me, thwarting my good intentions. But wait! There's good news also. Paul confidently asserts, "God is faithful, and He will not let you be tempted beyond your ability, but with the temptation He will also provide the way of escape, that you may be able to endure it" (1 Corinthians 10:13). Through medically-informed health education, your students will be equipped to make wise health decisions. Through health education that is shaped by the Scriptures, your students will be equipped by the Holy Spirit to make health decisions that also bring honor and praise to God their Savior. (6.4.1)

• Role-play someone who is being influenced to do something illegal. Ask a friend to role-play a person who is trying to convince the person not to get involved. Your friend should be sure to remind you of your Baptism and speak of Jesus' sacrifice for you on the cross as they encourage responsible, Christian behavior. After the role play, ask your class to discuss these questions: How do we influence each other concerning our health? Have we ever given each other unhealthy advice or provided an unhealthy influence? If yes, give examples and explain why the advice was unhealthy. Pray for the wisdom to provide healthy influences to others.
• Why do people get their bodies pierced or tattooed? What influences people to get tattoos? What are the health implications of these practices? Consider the body markings described or referred to in God's Word (Genesis 4:15; Leviticus 19:28; Ezekiel 9:4; John 19:33–37; Galatians 6:17). What mark does God place on us in Baptism? What does this mark mean to you? Write a devotion entitled "My Body—Marked for Christ."

Culture, Gender, and Age Differences and Health Practices

Today's classroom can be a virtual United Nations. Children are privileged to learn with others who have different backgrounds and faith foundations from their own. It is an opportunity for you as teacher to help the students in your classroom to learn to respectfully ask questions, explore life in many cultures, and share the Gospel of Jesus Christ. The United States Department for Substance Abuse and Mental Health Services Administration provides useful tips for teachers who work with students of various cultures at www.mentalhealth.samhsa.gov/cmhs/Emergency Services/culture.asp. People from cultures around the world have their own unique concepts about being healthy and proper health care. An informative summary of how various culture groups view health and health care is available from the gov-

• Relationships are very evident today in movies, television, and even school hallways. Choose a movie or television show, and identify the relationships that are featured. Describe the relationship, and give reasons why this relationship developed. What do the individuals do to show their love and care for each other? Is having sex a part of this relationship? How do the people help each other when things get tough? What threatens this relationship? Do you think this type of relationship is admired in our culture today? Do you think this relationship is God-pleasing or not? Is this relationship a good model for teens to follow? Explain your ideas. With your classmates, teacher, and parents, discuss this question: For Christian teens, what activities and attitudes indicate a wholesome relationship with others of the same

ernment of Queensland, Australia, at www.health.qld.gov.au/multicultural/cultdiv/default.asp. Use this resource to understand the health practices of various cultures, to provide information about these practices, and to understand the cultural background that may influence the health practices of your students and their families. Armed with these skills and information, you will be equipped to teach "for the sake of the gospel, that [you] may share with them in its blessings" (1 Corinthians 9:23). (6.4.2)

sex and with members of the opposite sex?
• How might culture, age, and gender influence what is eaten for breakfast? Make cartoon drawings that illustrate breakfast-eating patterns in various cultures, age levels, and genders. Are these breakfast-eating practices healthy? Do all the practices help people honor God with their bodies? Discuss your drawings, and place them on a bulletin board with a Scripture verse as the title.

Media, Influence on Health Practices

Our age is an age of media and readily available information. Commercials are everywhere. People seem to want instant communication. Increasingly sophisticated search engines enable us to locate huge amounts of information in seconds. All of this information helps to shape our attitudes. It would be easy to neglect God's Word, relegate it to an "only one of many" status, or think it irrelevant amid the authorities of the day. Since sin is the greatest threat to our physical and mental health, as Hezekiah well knew (Isaiah 38:16–17), God's pronouncement of the cure for sin through the suffering, death, and resurrection of His Son is the most important message the media and technologies of our day can help us proclaim. As you provide information about health practices and encourage young people to praise and honor God through the care and use of their bodies, may His Word be your most important tool. (6.4.3)

• Gather information regarding the types of health information you receive in commercials as you watch television during the week. What percentage of the information regarding health and beauty products focuses on beauty rather than health? Present your findings to your class. What attitudes toward the products are the commercials attempting to create? Whenever God provides healing or a way for us to care for our bodies, what response seems most appropriate (Matthew 15:30–31)?
• Use technology to make a health decision. Obtain a sound-level meter from an electronics supply store. Make a "How Loud Is Too Loud?" wheel following the directions that are available from the Oregon Museum of Science and Industry at www.dangerousdecibels.org/teachers_guide/DDB_TRG_Appendices_5.pdf. With the sound level meter, measure the loudness of sounds that you encounter during a typical day. Report your findings to your classmates, and show them how to use the sound-level meter. What sounds are too loud for healthy ears? Make recommendations for maintaining healthy ears. How are the suggested responses to loud sounds like "Turn it down," "Walk away," and "Protect your ears" similar to James's advice (James 1:21–27) and Peter's advice (1 Peter 5:6–10) concerning how to deal with any sin or temptation?

Health Needs, Special

You cannot judge a book by its cover! There are people who look perfectly normal (whatever standard that is) on the outside and yet are living with some tremendous difficulties on the inside. There are others who on the outside look as if they are very challenged and perhaps even lack basic skills yet possess minds and skills beyond expectation. Special health needs run the gamut from allergy medication to living with the help of a ventilator and a feeding tube. In Old Testament times, people with special needs were often considered outcasts and sinners, because people believed God would not have allowed such an illness to come to someone who practiced all the Jewish laws and rituals. For example, the disciples asked Jesus if the man born blind or his parents had sinned (John 9:2). Jesus set the record straight by responding that neither was the case, but that through the man's blindness the works of God would be displayed (John 9:1–5). A most important lesson to be learned as you teach to this standard is that people with special health needs are no less valuable than someone who appears whole. Both are God's creations, and both have been redeemed by Jesus. Both have gifts to offer families, friends, and the world. God uses each person to help and serve others. As you teach, nourish and capitalize on the opportunities children will have to learn important and unique things from one another, including how to care for each other's health and to respect each other as God's child. (6.4.4)

• Survey your classmates to see who uses special health-related equipment or assistance. If there are not many special needs identified, divide into groups and think about types of equipment that might be needed for protection. Think about the body's organ systems to give you ideas of what might stop working well and need special help. Did you include braces, glasses, casts, bike helmets, umbrellas, and football shoulder pads in your list? Who needs special help? What lessons did you learn from this process? How is Jesus' comment in Matthew 9:12–13 related to this discussion?

• Some may see it as a sad thing that a friend or family member has to use a walker or wheelchair. In reality, special equipment increases the number of things a person can do. Wheelchairs make it possible for people to coach, referee, and play basketball. Just as Monodnock frees those with special needs to do more things, the certainty of our forgiveness in Jesus' name frees us to do and be more because we no longer need to try to work our way into heaven.

HEALTH GOALS AND DECISION MAKING

INFORMATION BY TOPIC   DISCUSSION POINTS/ACTIVITIES

6.5   **Sixth-grade students in Lutheran schools will set goals and use decision-making skills to enhance their own health and the health of others.**

Health Decisions and Helpful Information

Have you ever drawn a conclusion about a specific person or event based on information passed on to you by someone else, only to discover a short time later that the information you were using was not accurate and made the conclusions you had reached incorrect? It is very important to use the latest and most accurate information available when making a decision. In health situations, seeking a second opinion is one way to avoid basing decisions on inadequate or inaccurately analyzed data. In trust relationships with God, the brief sentence, "Don't put a period where God has placed a comma" provides perspective. Of all the disciples, Peter seems to be a person who jumps before he looks. The Holy Spirit came to Peter and the disciples and made clear all that Jesus had told them (Acts 2:4). With this accurate and complete information, Peter, by God's grace, used his energy to evangelize others! What decisions are weighing heavily on you right now? Have you prayed to Jesus asking for His insight and wisdom? Have you talked with close and trusted faith-friends? As you make decisions, pray that God would provide for your every need in whatever lies before you. (6.5.1)

• Research and make a series of posters that illustrate the type of help each of these health specialists provides: dermatologists, optometrists, psychologists, orthodontists, oncologists, athletic trainers, and others of which you may have heard. In the Gospels, we read about people who, were they living today, would be seeing many of these specialists. Scripture tells us that Jesus healed people suffering from ailments that are treated by specialists today. What ailment did Jesus treat that health specialists can't treat (Matthew 9:2, 13; Mark 10:45; Luke 24:45–47; John 3:13–17; 20:30–31; Acts 4:8–12; Romans 3:23–24)? In an additional poster, praise Jesus for treating the ailment that you identified.

• How do families choose doctors? Ask your parents how the doctors your family consults were chosen. Ask your classmates to ask their parents for the same information. Compile your class information in a chart. Discuss the results of your survey. Which means of identifying a capable doctor seem most reliable to you? What would you do if, after your first visit, you felt that the physician you had chosen wasn't right for you? What are the benefits of having a family physician? In what ways is Jesus our model family physician (Psalm 103:1–3; Luke 18:15–17; Titus 3:5–7; Hebrews 4:14–16; 1 John 1:9)?

Decision-Making Process

Few decisions are set in concrete, but for some sixth graders, the tiniest decision can seem like a mountain to climb. Teaching decision-making skills, especially with regard to making health-related decisions, is good practice. The best practice of all in decision-making is to begin the process by heeding the advice of the hymn writer Joseph Scriven: "Take it to the Lord in prayer" from the hymn "What a Friend We Have in Jesus"

• Research decision-making processes at www.decide-guide.com/decision-step-models.html. With your classmates, discuss these questions: Should prayer be a part of every decision-making process? If so, when? Who is responsible for completing each step? Make a copy of your own decision-making model and keep it in an easily accessible place. In a small group, read through each of the steps and make certain everyone

(*LSB* 770, *LW* 516). God has promised to bless our decisions according to His purposes. "Commit your work to the LORD, and your plans will be established. The LORD has made everything for its purpose" (Proverbs 16:3–4). (6.5.2)

understands them. Use your decision-making model to decide an issue facing your class (e.g., where to go for a class picnic, which mission to support with an offering, a healthy menu for a grandparent's day breakfast). At what points in your decision-making effort did you pray? If necessary, modify your decision-making model to help your group and yourself improve your decision-making.

• What would you decide to do if someone you did not know contacted you online and asked for personal information? Go to www.4j.lane.edu/safety/rules.html, and print and read the guidelines developed for students in Oregon. Discuss this pledge with your classmates. How would following these guidelines increase your personal safety? In what ways do these guidelines help you live according to the Fourth Commandment? Thinking of yourself as God's baptized child, write your own pledge for online safety and share it with your parents and teachers.

Goals, Setting Health

Educators are forever setting goals for themselves and others—lesson plan goals, parent–student goals, individual goals to spend more time with family than with correcting papers. If you keep a day planner, do you block off space for "just me" time? Treat such time as you would any appointment; when people want to set a meeting at that time, you can honestly say that the time is already taken. Add a "family" and a "spouse" time as well. The goal is to devote time to your own physical and spiritual health. Use this standard to reach the goal of providing "just me" time for yourself. You have an excellent role model in Jesus, who made it a practice to spend time alone in prayer and thought—time that nourished Him for the days when He would give generously of His time for others. Because of His love for us, He took the time to give Himself for our salvation (Galatians 4:4). (6.5.3)

• Read this Web site to find out about foods that are good for you: tiki.oneworld.net/food/food_home.html. Find other Web sites that discuss the same topic, and compare the information provided. Summarize your findings for your class, and list foods that are good for you. Then, with several classmates, plan a menu for a picnic or meal that includes only foods that are good for you. Set a goal to increase the number of meals you eat that feature only foods that are good for you each week for the next two months. Keep records. At the end of two months report the results to your classmates. Reflect on the words of Jesus in Luke 14:28–32. What are the blessings of planning and working to reach a goal?

• Keep a sleep diary for a week; use the form at www.nhlbi.nih.gov/ health/public/sleep/starslp/teachers/sleep_diary.htm. Analyze the results. Meditate on Psalm 127:2. What is the psalmist's thought? An alternative translation of the last portion of this passage is "For He grants sleep to those He loves" (Psalm 127:2 NIV). What blessings does God give you as you sleep? Before you fall asleep at night, pray and sing one of the hymns in the "Evening" section of your hymnal.

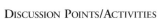

Recycling

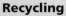

Reducing, reusing, and recycling—these may be nice sounding but rather empty words for some of us. We try to keep track of what goes in what bin or what one-sided scrap paper can be safely reused without unintentionally sharing personal information. Space is an issue for some whose living space is just not large enough to keep multiple containers going simultaneously. Where do you stand on the continuum? If you forget or just don't want to make the effort, do pangs of guilt come rushing over you? God placed the environment under the dominion of Adam and Eve in the garden. It, too, was spoiled by sin and awaits the final coming of Jesus Christ to become once again what it was made to be (Romans 8:18–23). As Adam's and Eve's heirs, we also have the responsibility to subdue and rule over the earth (Genesis 1:28), to work it and care for it (Genesis 2:15). As redeemed people of God through Jesus Christ, we are stewards of His creation and of the Gospel of salvation (1 Peter 4:9–11). By His grace, we are His children through faith in the Lord Jesus, stewards of His creation, and teachers of the Gospel who are privileged to proclaim the Good News to His people. (6.5.4)

• Working together in a small group, put your various skills to use to solve this riddle: How many trees might be saved during the time you are in grade school if you and your fellow class members used only recycled paper? Record the amount of paper recycled in one week by your class, predict the amount that will be recycled in a year, and then translate this figure into how many trees might be saved during the time you spend in elementary school. Some help to complete your project may be found at www.recycle.pdx.edu/pr_recycling101_fun_facts.php. When you complete your project, meditate on this thought: We may work hard to save trees. What did Jesus do to save us (Romans 4:25; 1 Corinthians 15:3–4; 1 Peter 1:18–20)?

• Read Romans 8:18–23. How is all of creation in "bondage to decay" (Romans 8:21)? What will happen to all of creation when the children of God receive His glory on the Last Day? What encouragement and comfort does this insight bring to you? In love, God will one day restore all of creation. How is this teaching related to being reducers, reusers, and recyclers? Plan a way that you and your classmates can help restore the beauty of God's creation near where you live.

HEALTH COMMUNICATION AND OTHER SKILLS

6.6   **Sixth-grade students in Lutheran schools will develop the interpersonal communication and other skills to better their own and others' health.**

Communicating Feelings

In Jesus' day, people who wanted His help boldly used both verbal and nonverbal communication to make their needs known. When a blind beggar near Jericho (Luke 18:35–43) heard a large crowd passing by, he asked what was happening. When he was told that Jesus of Nazareth was passing by, the man cried out, "Jesus, Son of David, have mercy on me!" (Luke 18:38). Even though people did not want him to use his verbal skills, he doggedly used them to communicate his feelings, wants, and needs. In mercy, Jesus healed him. In another instance, a man who was deaf and who also had a speech impediment was brought to Jesus (Mark 7:31–37). The people who brought the man to Jesus begged Him to heal the man. The man himself could only use nonverbal skills to indicate his need. Jesus, in turn, first used nonverbal sign language and then spoke: "Ephphatha," which means "Be opened!" Verbally, only one word was spoken by Jesus, yet the man was immediately able both to hear and speak plainly. Jesus had given the man verbal skills. Jesus' command can be our prayer. Pray, "Lord, open my heart, that I might hear and receive your gifts in faith. Lord, open the ears and eyes of my students, that they might understand Your love for them and carry it beyond this room in verbal and nonverbal ways." Some ideas and resources for helping students express themselves appropriately are available at www.cccoe.net/social/expressfeelings.htm. (6.6.1)

• Write a short story about a fictional character who experienced a bad storm or similar event. Tell how this character felt and what he or she did to deal with various difficulties. Let the character tell about a Bible passage that was especially helpful in this situation. Toward the end of your story, let the character tell what he or she learned from the experience. Share your story with your class.

• With a classmate, plan a puppet play in which two characters arrive in the lunch line at the same time, get to the water fountain at the same time, or get to a favorite bus seat at the same time. Make several bag puppets to use in your skit. Plan that these characters will get into an argument about who goes first and that the argument gets rather heated. At the height of the argument, stop. Ask your classmates these questions: How did each character feel? What did each one want? How could this conflict be resolved? Ask one pair of volunteers to enact a lose-lose solution; everyone is a loser. Ask another set of volunteers to enact a lose-win situation; one character clearly gets the better deal from the situation. Ask another set of volunteers to enact a win-win solution where everyone receives something of what they want. To conclude this activity, read Psalm 34:11–14, discuss the ideas of the psalmist, and pray that you and your classmates may pursue peace in each tense situation. Jesus came to bring peace to us (John 14:27; 16:33). Through His death and resurrection, we have peace with God and each other (Romans 5:1; Ephesians 2:13–22).

Communicating Care and Respect

How has God communicated His care, respect, and consideration for people, His creation, throughout the centuries? What means has He used to show His love? Recall these: He provided clothing for Adam and Eve and marked Cain so no

• Create an activity that will show care, respect, and consideration for someone in your community. For example, interact in some way with your church's homebound members. Ask your pastor or teacher to identify people you might visit and to

INFORMATION BY TOPIC

one would hurt him. Rather than allow His plan and His promise to be destroyed in a flood of evil, He destroyed the evil and preserved Noah, his family, His promise of a Savior, and a rich array of animals in the waters of the great flood; in our Baptism, He similarly drowns evil and preserves us for eternal life by washing us clean of all sin. He sent His own Son to be punished and die on the cross for our sin and raised Him to new life, and through His Son, He gives us new life. In His Word, He gives us the good news of the Gospel. In the Lord's Supper, He nourishes us with His body and blood that is coupled with the words of forgiveness in Christ. Remind your students of the many ways God communicates His love and care for us. (6.6.2)

DISCUSSION POINTS/ACTIVITIES

help you to arrange the visit. Ahead of time, prepare and laminate bookmarks that have Bible verses on them or grow plants in decorated pots. Plan to sing songs, read the newspaper or a story, and present the gifts you prepared. Close your visit with a short devotion.

• Plan a way to thank others for the care and consideration they show to others. Take candid photographs of people demonstrating care, respect, and consideration for others. Use your pictures to create a slide show, or place your pictures on poster board and display the posters in your church or school. Include music if you'd like. Thank God for these people in your presentation. Praise Him for the love He has shown us by giving His Son, Jesus, to be our Savior. Only because Jesus first loved us are we able to love others (1 John 4:10–11, 19).

Responsibility

Most of us wear many hats in our lives. Right now you are reading this with the head covering of a teacher. This calling comes with its unique responsibilities. As a teacher, you educate a large number of children, and your influence will be felt throughout their lives. What a child learns from you helps mold a developing conscience, an ethical life, a moral code, and an awareness of how very much each one is loved by God through Jesus Christ. Your influence cannot be measured. You have an impact on how the children will interact with one another, siblings, and parents. In turn, each of your students will influence their own children and associates. So you have a huge responsibility, and that's in only one area of your life. Thanks be to God that you do not have to carry this responsibility all on your own! Your coworkers and principal and your student's parents and families all help shoulder the burden and the joy. Take time to look at your own personal responsibilities. Are they clearly referenced in your personal mission statement? What are the characteristics of a responsible person? Never forget that the master teacher, Jesus Christ Himself, promises to equip you for and help you fulfill the responsibilities He has given you. His promise is that He will be with

• As you grow and mature, increasing responsibilities are often an issue. Some responsibilities you are given. Some you assume on your own. Some you have, but you don't necessarily want them. Some you would like to have but can't have them or aren't given them. Divide a piece of paper into four sections, and label each section with a heading indicating each of these types of responsibility: "Given Responsibilities," "Assumed Responsibilities," "Unwanted Responsibilities," and "Wanted but Denied Responsibilities." Write examples of each type of responsibility in the appropriate box. Think about responsibilities you have for your own clothes, health, learning, and safety. Compare your responses with those of your classmates. Are your responsibilities much different from those of your classmates? What might be the reasons you are denied some responsibilities? Sixth graders are often called upon to watch out for a younger sibling until the parents arrive home from work. Think back to the story of baby Moses and his sister Miriam. How did Miriam show that she was a responsible and quick-thinking person while watching out for her little brother (Exodus 2:1–10)? How did Jesus feel about the responsibility of adults toward young children (Luke

you (Matthew 28:20) and will send His Spirit to be with you to pray for you (Romans 8:26) and to give you the words you need and the manner to say them (Mark 13:11; Acts 1:8). Thanks be to God! Some useful ideas for teaching responsibility are available at www.goodcharacter.com/YCC/BeingResponsible.html.(6.6.3)

18:15–17)? What chores or responsibilities have been given to you? Which ones are health-related? On a scale of one (I don't carry out this responsibility well at all.) to four (I am very responsible in this respect.), how would you rate yourself in carrying out the responsibilities listed on your chart? Ask God to help you be more responsible as you plan how to improve in the areas that you identified.

• Take a survey of your classmates. Ask them this question: What responsibilities do friends have toward their friends? List all the ideas presented. Group similar ideas. Create a set of posters depicting the three or four most mentioned ideas. What did Jesus do for His friends (Psalm 25:14; John 15:13–14)? Use one poster to tell how Jesus is a friend to each person.

Listening Skills

There is one thing of which we can be sure: God has good listening skills. When Israel was enslaved in Egypt, "During those many days the king of Egypt died, and the people of Israel groaned because of their slavery and cried out for help. Their cry for rescue from slavery came up to God. And God heard their groaning, and God remembered His covenant with Abraham, with Isaac, and with Jacob. God saw the people of Israel—and God knew" (Exodus 2:23–25). He hears grumbling (Exodus 16:9, 12). He hears the cries of the needy (Exodus 22:27). He hears the pleas of His servants (2 Kings 19:14–37). He hears the remorse of the repentant heart (Psalm 51:1–7). Only on Calvary, when His own Son pleaded for mercy, did He seemingly not hear a prayer so that we might have salvation (Matthew 27:46–50). Through the sacrifice of His Son, God reestablished our relationship with Him as His people, His heirs of eternal glory (Titus 3:4–7). (6.6.4)

• We don't listen with our ears only. Every aspect of our body from the top of our head to the bottom of our feet plays a role in letting the speaker know how actively involved and interested we are in what is said. This type of listening is called active listening. Observe this type of listening as you do the following activity. Ask your teacher to arrange a time when you can read a story to a group of younger students. Practice reading the story before you read to them. When you read, notice how students react. Do they ask questions? imitate sounds? act out the actions? They are actively listening. When we listen actively, we learn. Was Jesus a passive or active listener in these stories: John 4:7– 42; 8:1–11; 10:22–39? Were the people listening to Jesus passive or active listeners? Jesus listened so actively to us in our need that He took our place on the cross to die for the sins of the world (John 3:16).

• Select an article about healthy feet from a resource such as www.foot.com/. Prepare to read it to your class. To prepare your classmates to learn from your reading, briefly give your classmates an overview of what you will read. Then show them a diagram or picture and tell them about the organization of the article. Alert your classmates to listen for the two or three main ideas in the reading; perhaps provide a short fill-in outline or set of fill-in sentences that will help them remember the main ideas. Prepare one or two discussion questions to consider at the end of your reading. To close your presentation, tell about a Bible passage relating to feet that shows that God faithfully gives secure footing to His people, especially through Jesus, His Son and our Savior. Use a concordance to find such passages; some to consider include Psalm 18:33; 40:1–2; and 56:13. Arrange with your teacher for a time to present your reading.

Negotiation Skills

The activities associated with this standard suggest the use of "I" messages to communicate anger. Some useful teaching activities to help students distinguish between passive, aggressive, and assertive statements and to use assertive behaviors appropriately are available at www.sasked.gov.sk.ca/docs/health/health6-9/g7append.html#f. As we teach assertive behavior and conversation skills to sixth graders, we are adding a number of healthy items to their tool box of life. Jesus used "I" messages. Do you recall a few of them, such as "I am the Bread of Life" and "I am the Good Shepherd"? These messages echo God's statement to Moses at the burning bush. Moses wanted to know what he should tell the people about God. God responded, "I AM WHO I AM" (Exodus 3:14). So as Jesus continued in His ministry and named Himself with the beginning "I am," He was again drawing attention to His relationship with Yahweh. May the great I AM guide and bless you as you help your students practice and make their own the power of assertive refusal both in their interactions with people and with those who attempt to deceive and lead them astray from the one true God and Father of our Lord, Jesus Christ. (6.6.5)

• Think of several times when you did not approve of something or felt uncomfortable. You wanted to say something but didn't know what to say. Fill in these model sentences to practice thinking what you could say.
When you stop (identify the behavior that you don't like or approve of) I will be able to help you

_____.

I understand that you're upset about this. When you can talk without (shouting, being disrespectful), I'll be willing to discuss _____.
You can do _____as soon as you

_____.

Write sentences for several situations, and read them aloud to yourself or to a partner. In your sentences, refer to your Christian beliefs and practices that come from God's Word. Be ready to walk away from a harmful situation until there is a better, safer time for discussion and problem-solving.
• Do you believe you have to say "Yes" all the time to be liked? You have a right to say "No." How would you say no in the following situations? Role-play saying no in each of the following situations: (1) Your friends ask you to go to a show that you don't want to see. (2) A boy or girl that you don't particularly like wants to hold hands with you. (3) A person you hang out with asks to see your homework so he or she can copy it. (4) Your family is watching your favorite TV show, but you have tons of homework. Role-play several situations you create. Then think about James's advice to Christian people who were attempting to live

lives that praised their Savior: "Above all, my brothers, do not swear, either by heaven or by earth or by any other oath, but let your 'yes' be yes and your 'no' be no, so that you may not fall under condemnation" (James 5:12). Remember also that you are God's child, loved so much that His Son gave His life to save you (1 John 4:9–10).

Conflict, Causes and Resolution of

Ever since Eve listened to that snake and believed the devil's wily tale, sin entered the world, and with it came a whole host of problems (Genesis 3). Originally there existed no conflict in the Garden of Eden, but following the fall conflict became part of human existence. There was conflict with God as well as with other human beings. What is truly amazing, for Adam and Eve as well as for us today, is that even though the first couple tried hiding from God and skipping out on His usual evening walk with them, He still sought them out and talked about what had happened. God set down the consequences of their choice, and He showed them great grace by promising a Savior to come (Genesis 3:15). He also provided for their needs outside of the garden. Many adolescents will face conflict situations. Often they will not remember why or how the conflict began. To complicate matters, the manner in which boys and girls settle conflict is quite different. Talk with your class about the origin of sin and its continued effect on us today. Be certain to talk about the grace and mercy of God upon His children, through His Son, Jesus Christ. Our Savior's journey involved constant confrontations with Satan, the father of lies, but on the cross He won the victory over sin, death, and Satan. Through the forgiveness of sin won by Jesus Christ on the cross, we have peace with God (John 16:33; Romans 5:1). In Him is the foundation that people have for peace with each other (Ephesians 2). (6.6.6)

• Since you have been in school, it is quite likely that you have been in an argument. You may have been the initiator of conflict or the one on the receiving end. Both are uncomfortable positions. There is also the possibility that you have been encouraged to take sides in an argument. Conflict is not strange to you. With your classmates, brainstorm possible causes of conflict between people. Draw from your own experience, but do not use actual names. Discuss these questions: What is the root cause of conflict among all people, not just adolescents (Matthew 15:19; Romans 5:12; 8:7; 1 John 3:8)? What grace and mercy did God show to people to help settle the conflicts among us (Galatians 3:13; Colossians 1:13–14)? What did Jesus call His disciples to do in order to resolve conflict among them (Matthew 20:20–28)? How does His call apply to us today?

• Conflict can grow and breed one new strand after another. Sometimes the individuals involved are so closely related to the problem that they need help to see the issues more clearly. This help may come in the form of a peer mediator, principal, pastor, or teacher. Read and study the section entitled "Confession" in Luther's Small Catechism. Study also "A Short Form of Confession." Write a paper about how following a form of Confession and Absolution would be useful in helping to bring reconciliation to a conflict.

HEALTH ADVOCACY

6.7   **Sixth-grade students in Lutheran schools will develop the ability to advocate for healthy lifestyles for themselves, their family, and the community.**

Information, Reliability of

Over the centuries, people have believed a great deal of dubious information about the causes of health problems and the cures for them. It is interesting to browse through a farmers' almanac or memoirs of those who settled our country to find the remedies for illness that were used. A favorite show on cable television called *The Mythbusters* sometimes takes on the task of proving or disproving health remedies that have long been held as fact. News specials frequently do the same type of debunking of health-care myths. There are reliable old home remedies and there are the snake-oil remedies. One illness everyone suffers is sin-sickness. Here too, many ideas have been proposed for relieving this disorder. Many people choose to use do-it-yourself remedies that cannot provide any type of help or healing. Sin-sickness is only taken away by confessing our sins and receiving forgiveness, or absolution, from Jesus, our Lord and Savior. Faithful use of Luther's "Short Form for Confession" or a similar form would certainly be a healthy lifestyle change to advocate! Look for more contemporary forms of Confession in your hymnal. Proclaim God's Law to produce Confession. Tell the great Good News of Jesus, the physician and healer of all, and announce His Absolution to the repentant. This is spiritual health teaching at its best. (6.7.1)

• Just because information is written down and sounds accurate does not guarantee that it will be accurate. Just because a tune or a phrase seems catchy and useful does not mean that it will contain valid medical advice for everyone. With your classmates, identify several clever or not-so-clever health product advertisements you have seen. As a group, choose the five you feel are the most effective strategies. Develop a survey form, and survey students in your school to find out which of the five ads the students think communicates health information most accurately. Total the results, and rank the advertisements in order. Next, examine the health information content of each advertisement. Rank the ads from most information to least information. Compare the results of the survey with the study of the ad content. Are students in your school able to determine if advertisements contain valuable health information? Do you think students in your school think much about the advertising they see and hear? Several apostles advise us to examine the spiritual messages we receive to test every teaching to make sure it is in accord with God's Word (Romans 12:2; 1 Thessalonians 5:20–21; 1 John 4:1–3). Similarly, it is best to examine carefully the health information we receive and to compare it with information prepared by reputable scholars before we follow the advice or use the medication. Report your findings and make recommendations to your fellow students by writing a newsletter article.

• Work with your classmates in a small group to prepare an interesting advertisement that contains much reliable information about a food or health product. Provide information about the health benefits of the product. Your advertisement can be designed as a PowerPoint presentation, a poster, a sign, a skit, a TV ad, or an announcement. Present your advertisement to your class. Use the same technique to advertise the Gospel of Jesus Christ in your community. Present your advertisement to your class. Discuss: Why is presenting the Gospel accurately just as important as presenting

INFORMATION BY TOPIC

DISCUSSION POINTS/ACTIVITIES

health information accurately?

• Write a letter to the editor of your town's newspaper or create a proposal for a change needed in your community that would promote healthy living. Present it to the town council's forum. Find out what procedure to follow in order to do this. Discuss this question with your classmates: If the evangelists of the Early Christian Church had this type of media at their disposal, how do you think they might have used it?

Choices, Supporting Others

God created us to live in community with one another. He created Eve to be a companion for Adam. He placed them in charge of the garden and commanded them to be fruitful and multiply (Genesis 1:26–31; 2:18–25). He talked with them. He wanted them to have close relationships with each other and with Him. When Adam and Eve fell into sin, God immediately set into motion His plan to reestablish that relationship with His creation through the sacrifice of His Son (Genesis 3:15). One key to being able to equip students to make wise health choices is to work to establish community and trust in your classroom. One of the great blessings of Lutheran schools is that we have the opportunity to help and care for one another in Christ. Help your students build relationships with classmates, siblings, and their extended family so they will be at ease when they need help in making important health decisions and when they reach out into the community at large with the love and care of Jesus and the message of salvation He secured. (6.7.2)

• David and Jonathan, Ruth and Naomi, David and Nathan, Paul and Timothy—one thing these pairs all have in common is that they supported and encouraged one another; they enjoyed strong and trusting relationships. Each of these was also able to help others with choices that had to be made. Consult your Bible and identify the choices that each of the groups of people helped each other make. Discuss these questions with your classmates: How did the people help each other? How did Christ help us (1 Corinthians 15:3; 1 John 2:2)?

• Suppose a friend of yours mentions that he or she is thinking about smoking cigarettes. How would you go about helping that person make a decision that is best for his or her health? List as many things that could be done as you can. Ask your classmates to help you compile your list. Mark the ones you can do immediately with a checkmark. Mark the ones that will take some time to do with a triangle. Mark the ones that probably need to be done by a health-care professional with a circle. Mark the ones that are related to a teaching of Scripture with a cross. Write a short article for your school newspaper entitled "Helping Your Friends Decide about Smoking."

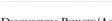

Community Agencies

We usually think of asking Jesus for help as He invited us to do (Matthew 11:28). But can you think of instances when Jesus pointed His disciples or others to go to someone in the community for help? He sent His disciples to tell others the "kingdom of heaven is at hand" (Matthew 10:7) and to depend on people in the community for their hospitality (Matthew 10:9–11). He directed His disciples to "Go into the village" to find a donkey for His use (Matthew 21:2). Another time He told His disciples to "Go into the city" to arrange for the use of a room to celebrate the Passover (Matthew 26:18). He Himself stayed at the home of Mary, Martha, and Lazarus (John 12:1–2). Predominantly in Scripture, we see Jesus feeding, healing, and helping others. He came to seek and save the lost and did so with His death on the cross and His resurrection to new life. But Jesus knew and used the community resources available to Him. His life is a model for Christian educators in this respect also. Our mission, and the predominant mission of Lutheran schools, is to bring the good news of the Gospel to others, but we also use the resources of our communities when they can be of service to the people in our care. Using community specialists, facilities, and speakers can enrich the lives of our students and families. As we do so, we point our students and families to resources, especially health resources, they can use to meet their needs. (6.7.3)

• With your classmates, compile a list of community health agencies and resources that your families use or that are available to help children and families. Have each student find out information about one of the resources and prepare a poster advertising the services of the agency or resource. Display your posters in your building to inform people about these community resources. Make a banner to provide a theme for your display. Use the slogan "God's Gifts for Healthy Living" or a similar one.

• Collect the calendars that list the community health-education programs of agencies in your community. Libraries, hospitals, the Red Cross, and county and state government agencies often plan such activities and prepare calendars. From the calendars, select the health programs that would be of most interest and benefit to students in your school and families in your congregation. Make a calendar that lists these activities and the time and place when the activity will be held. Place this Bible passage on your calendar: "I will restore health to you . . . declares the LORD" (Jeremiah 30:17).

• Invite a parish nurse or a member of your congregation who is a health-care professional to speak to your class. Or invite a fire safety person or a representative from a local utility, such as the electric company or the gas company, to speak to your class. Ask the person to speak to your class about safety, the proper care of our bodies, and about places to go for help in your community. Ask how your class can help promote the health and safety of people in the community. Volunteer to help others sponsor a bloodmobile visit to your congregation or conduct a health fair. In this way, you will be following in the footsteps of Jesus, who not only healed the wounds of our sins by His death on the cross but who also healed many people.

Goals, Cooperation to Achieve

To encourage the Church and God's people to work together cooperatively, the apostle Paul used the imagery of the parts of the body working together (1 Corinthians 12:12–31; Ephesians 4:1–16), each doing its part without being jealous of what another part could do. Each person has gifts and abilities that are unique, and yet the gifts are necessary to the successful functioning of the Church in its efforts to proclaim the message of salvation in Jesus Christ to all people. When illness or accident causes one part of the body to lose its ability to function, disciplined training and relearning takes place. New nerve pathways are developed through therapy and practice. Clear goals are set so that the body may again work together. The part that is weaker may be aided by a stronger part (1 Corinthians 12:21–26). The cooperative working together of the body that God made is one of the great blessings of His creation. When, through sin, we lost our ability to function as God's people (Ephesians 4:14), He restored us through the life and death of His Son (Ephesians 2:13). Through the Spirit, He strengthens us for service and praise. Praise be to God for His gifts. Thanks be to Jesus for taking on our human form and giving His life for ours. Thanks be to the Holy Spirit who serves as advocate and counselor, translator and motivator. All thanks to God now and forever. (6.7.4)

• We all have goals. Perhaps they are not all clearly defined, but at least we have a general knowledge of what we would like to be able to do in a given length of time. Name a health goal you would like to reach in the next several months. It may be to run a six- or seven-minute mile, to brush your teeth regularly after lunch, or to eat more fruits and fewer candies. Discuss your goal with a family member or friend and ask them to help you reach your goal by reminding you of your goal and, perhaps, by being your partner as you work to reach the goal. Read together Paul's words in Philippians 3:12–17 and discuss these questions: What was Paul's goal? Who did he want to join him in working toward his goal? What were to be the blessings of working toward his goal? With your partner, create a chart or calendar that describes intermediate goals for you to reach. Keep records of what you do. Reward yourselves when you reach your goal. Thank God for the blessings He gives to you as you work together.

• Ask your family to make it a goal to take part in a cooperative effort once or twice a year to help others in your community or church who need additional assistance to live a more joyful or complete life. Your family could offer to provide transportation to doctor's appointments or write letters for a shut-in, volunteer at a local food bank, or offer to do childcare for parents who meet together for Bible study or participate in an exercise class. Place a large star on your family's calendar each time you help someone in the community. Remember that you are the hands and feet of Jesus, doing His caring work as you serve.

CHAPTER 6

Topics in Health Education for Lutheran Educators

The three articles that follow give information about eating disturbances, allergies, and school policies. These topics directly affect many children today. The emotional health and physical health of children are interrelated, and both, as is true of all aspects of life, are affected by one's spiritual health. Our concern about health is led by our Savior's example, as He time and again felt compassion for those in need and helped them. He calls on us to show compassion and care too. Galatians 6:10 says to us, "As we have opportunity, let us do good to everyone, and especially to those who are of the household of faith." Let us respond to the needs of the children in our schools and in our care not only as created children of God, but also as redeemed and sanctified believers in Christ.

Healthy Eating— The Key to a Healthy Body Image

According to the latest government figures, more youngsters than ever (10 percent) are overweight, and between 16 and 33 percent of them are obese. On the other side of the weight issue, some youngsters become so preoccupied with being thin that they develop eating disorders (estimated seven million girls and one million boys). It's easier to prevent problems than to manage them later when they occur. The key to preventing both kinds of eating disturbances is instilling healthy eating and exercise habits at a young age.

How to Help

• Lead by example. Research shows that children imitate their parents' behavior. If you make an effort to maintain a healthy attitude and healthy eating habits, your children are more likely to do the same now and for the rest their lives.

• Come to terms with your own food issues and body image. Take a look at your own food habits and ideas about weight. Your comments and ideas about appearance can influence what your children think is acceptable or desirable. How many times have you heard yourself make a negative comment about how you look in an outfit? "Do I look fat in this?" or "Boy! These jeans make my thighs look fat!" Kids are listening and take in that a person is valued by his or her appearance.

• Give up dieting—it doesn't work! What's a healthy weight? Check with your doctor to understand how your child compares to established standards for height and weight.

How to Calculate Your BMI (Body Mass Index)

Multiply your weight in pounds by 703; divide by height in inches; divide again by height in inches, and the result is your BMI. For example, a thirteen-year-old boy who weighs 190 pounds and is 5′5″ tall would have a BMI=190 x 703 ÷ 65 ÷ 65 = 31.6, indicating that he is obese. A healthy BMI is between 18.5 and 24.9.

Start with Small Changes

• Cut back on soda and juice.

• Switch to skim milk. (Kids don't need as much milk as the dairy industry recommends.)

• Substitute fruit for dessert.

• Drink eight to eleven 8-ounce glasses of water daily.

• Rather than make a particular food taboo, use it in moderation for treats.

• Work towards following the federal dietary guidelines.

Healthy Eating—Some Dos

- Eat breakfast.
- Eat five to six small meals/snacks daily.
- Eat slowly and stop eating when you're satisfied.
- Eat when you're hungry.
- Eat together as a family.
- Have plenty of healthy snacks available.
- Make fast food only an occasional treat.

Healthy Eating—Some Don'ts

- Put your child on a restrictive diet.
- Skip meals.
- Use food as a reward or a comfort. (Substitute a special trip, art or sports supplies, movie, etc., as a reward.)
- Withhold food as punishment.
- Eat in front of the television.
- Force children to eat when they're not hungry.

Get Active

- Aim for thirty to sixty minutes of moderate physical activity daily.
- Encourage walking, biking, swimming, skating, ball sports, and so on.
- Reduce your child's total television screen time to less than two hours daily.

Body Image—What Is It?

Body image is how you think and feel about your body. It may have nothing to do with actual appearance. Each person holds an image of the perfect body and evaluates his/her appearance against this ideal. Poor body image can lead to eating disorders, depression, and low self-esteem.

Helping Children Develop a Healthy Body Image

- Foster a strong sense of identity and self-worth by letting your child know she is loved and appreciated whatever her weight.
- Focus on health and positive qualities, not weight.
- Be involved in your child's life and praise her for her accomplishments.
- Notice the contradictory messages from the media, and help children critique them. Help children understand that the "ideals" portrayed in fashion magazines are unrealistic and absurdly out of line with what a real body looks like. (Studies show that by age 17 a child has received over 250,000 commercial messages, and 50 percent of commercials aimed at girls focused on physical attractiveness.)
- Talk openly about ads, articles, Web sites or window displays that promote either eating disorders or unhealthy body image.
- Never tease a child about his looks, weight, or body shape.
- Encourage expressions of individuality. Teach children to appreciate people for who they are, rather than what they look like.
- Make your child feel he has an important role in the family by assigning age-appropriate household tasks.
- Celebrate diversity.
- Watch for "fat talk," such as "good" or "bad" foods, among yourself and others.

Eating Disorders

Eating disorders may occur when a person's preoccupation with food and weight becomes obsessive and results in starvation, overeating, and purging to a degree that becomes dangerous. Eating disorders can limit other aspects of a person's life and can seriously affect physical and mental health. Following are the most common types of eating disorders:

- Anorexia nervosa is a serious and life-threatening disorder which is usually due to emotional issues. People with anorexia nervosa have an intense fear of getting fat, even when underweight. They are generally obsessed with food, but deny their hunger and starve themselves. Many also limit other aspects of their lives such as relationships and social activities or pleasures. Anorexia can start as a desire to lose weight and a need to maintain control.

- Bulimia nervosa, a related and serious disorder with medical consequences, is harder to detect. It refers to a cycle of out-of-control eating followed by some form of purging, such as self-induced vomiting, excessive use of laxatives, or obsessive exercising. Individuals with bulimia may have other out-of-control behaviors, such as spending money, abusing drugs or alcohol, or chaotic relationships.

- Binge eating disorder is characterized by episodes of compulsive overeating followed by periods of guilt and depression.

Warning Signs

Anorexia Nervosa

- Excessive weight loss—15 percent or more of ideal body weight

- Distorted body image—feels fat even if thin

- Food rituals

- Lack of menstrual cycles

- Fine hair on face, arms and torso

- Wearing baggy clothing

- Vigorous exercise at odd hours

- Paleness, dizziness, fainting spells

- Repeated attempts at dieting

- Self-conscious or embarrassed about eating

- Perfectionism

- Eating for emotional comfort

Bulimia Nervosa

- Missing food/secretive eating

- Fluctuating weight (10–15 pounds)

- Cuts/scrapes on back of hand from when fingers are pushed down the throat to induce vomiting

- Tooth decay

- Uses bathroom after meals

- Diet pills/laxative abuse

- Self-disparagement related to food intake

- Swollen glands, puffy cheeks, broken blood vessels under the eyes

- Reacts to emotional stress by eating

Binge Eating

- Eating large amounts of food when not hungry

- Eating very rapidly until the point of feeling uncomfortably full

- Often eating alone due to shame or embarrassment

- Feeling depressed, disgusted, or guilty after eating

- Marked weight fluctuations

How Parents Can Help

A child with an eating disorder may be reluctant to acknowledge the problem. Let him/her know you care and want to help.

- Be aware of your own reactions and prejudices about people's weight.

- Realize that you can support your child, but you cannot control her eating.

- Do not discuss weight, appearance, or food intake.

- Watch for signs that physical and/or emotional health are worsening.

- Don't compare him to others or make comments about his appearance.

- Contact your pediatrician or family doctor and ask for referrals to a psychiatrist, therapist, and nutritionist.

About the Author

Melissa Nishawala, MD, is Assistant Professor of Psychiatry at the NYU School of Medicine and the Director of the Tisch Young Adult Program at the NYU Child Study Center. Dr. Nishawala's special interests are in eating disorders and autism spectrum disorders.

Written by and reprinted with permission from the NYU Child Study Center. Further information is available from their Web site (www.about ourkids.org).

School Guidelines for Managing Students with Food Allergies

Food allergies can be life threatening. The risk of accidental exposure to foods can be reduced in the school setting if schools work with students, parents, and physicians to minimize risks and provide a safe educational environment for food-allergic students.

Family's Responsibility

• Notify the school of the child's allergies.

• Work with the school team to develop a plan that accommodates the child's needs throughout the school, including in the classroom, in the cafeteria, in after-care programs, during school-sponsored activities, and on the school bus, as well as developing a Food Allergy Action Plan.

• Provide written medical documentation, instructions, and medications as directed by a physician, using the Food Allergy Action Plan as a guide. Include a photo of the child on the written form.

• Provide properly labeled medications and replace medications after use or upon expiration.

• Educate the child in the self-management of food allergies including safe and unsafe foods; strategies for avoiding exposure to unsafe foods; symptoms of allergic reactions; how and when to tell an adult they may be having an allergy-related problem; and how to read food labels (age appropriate).

• Review policies/procedures with the school staff, the child's physician, and the child (if age appropriate) after a reaction has occurred.

• Provide emergency contact information.

School's Responsibility

• Be knowledgeable about and follow applicable federal laws including ADA, IDEA, Section 504, and FERPA and any state laws or district policies that apply.

• Review the health records submitted by parents and physicians.

• Include food-allergic students in school activities. Students should not be excluded from school activities solely based on their food allergy.

• Identify a core team of, but not limited to, a school nurse, teacher, principal, school food service and nutrition manager/director, and counselor (if available) to work with parents and the student (age appropriate) to establish a prevention plan. Changes to the prevention plan to promote food allergy management should be made with core team participation.

• Assure that all staff who interact with the student on a regular basis understand the food allergy, can recognize symptoms, know what to do in an emergency, and work with other school staff to eliminate the use of food allergens in the allergic student's meals, educational tools, arts and crafts projects, or incentives.

• Practice the Food Allergy Action Plans before an allergic reaction occurs to assure the efficiency/effectiveness of the plans.

• Coordinate with the school nurse to be sure medications are appropriately stored and that an emergency kit is available that contains a physician's standing order for epinephrine. In states where regulations permit, medications are kept in an easily accessible secure location central to designated school personnel, not in locked cupboards or drawers. Students should be allowed to carry their own epinephrine, if age appropriate, after approval from the students' physician/clinic, parent, and school nurse, and allowed by state or local regulations.

• Designate school personnel who are properly trained to administer medications in accordance with the state nursing and Good Samaritan laws governing the administration of emergency medications.

• Be prepared to handle a reaction, and ensure that there is a staff member available who is properly trained to administer medications during the school day regardless of time or location.

- Review policies/prevention plan with the core team members, parents/guardians, student (age appropriate), and physician after a reaction has occurred.

- Work with the district transportation administrator to assure that school bus driver training includes symptom awareness and what to do if a reaction occurs.

- Recommend that all buses have communication devices in case of an emergency.

- Enforce a "no eating" policy on school buses with exceptions made only to accommodate special needs under federal or similar laws or school district policy. Discuss appropriate management of food allergy with family.

- Discuss field trips with the family of the food-allergic child to decide appropriate strategies for managing the food allergy.

- Follow federal/state/district laws and regulations regarding sharing medical information about the student.

- Take threats or harassment against an allergic child seriously.

Student's Responsibility

- Should not trade food with others

- Should not eat anything with unknown ingredients or known to contain any allergen

- Should be proactive in the care and management of their food allergies and reactions based on their developmental level

- Should notify an adult immediately if they eat something they believe may contain the food to which they are allergic

More detailed suggestions for implementing these objectives and creating a specific plan for each individual student in order to address his or her particular needs are available in The Food Allergy & Anaphylaxis Network's (FAAN) School Food Allergy Program. The School Food Allergy Program has been endorsed and/or supported by the Anaphylaxis Committee of the American Academy of Allergy Asthma and Immunology, the National Association of School Nurses, and the Executive Committee of the Section on

Allergy and Immunology of the American Academy of Pediatrics. FAAN can be reached at 800/929-4040.

The following organizations participated in the development of this document:

American School Food Service Association

National Association of Elementary School Principals

National Association of School Nurses

National School Boards Association

The Food Allergy & Anaphylaxis Network.

Reprinted with permission from The Food Allergy & Anaphylaxis Network.

A Model School Wellness Policy, Emphasizing Physical Activity and Nutrition

The following is a compilation of ideas for a wellness policy for a school. It includes wide-ranging possibilities that you may choose to adapt, add to, or delete. (Note: The name chosen for this sample school is St. Luke because Luke the apostle was a physician concerned about health.)

Preamble

Whereas, God's Word speaks of our bodies as temples of the Holy Spirit (1 Corinthians 3:16) and as being bought with the price of Christ's own blood (1 Corinthians 6:19–20);

Whereas, God's Word also admonishes us to "present yourselves to God as those who have been brought from death to life, and your members to God as instruments for righteousness" (Romans 6:13);

Whereas, God's Word also tells us that "whether you eat or drink, or whatever you do, do all to the glory of God" (1 Corinthians 10:31);

Whereas, these imperatives from God's Word encourage us to think of our bodies as His gifts to us and His place to reside and to use our bodies to bring honor and glory to Him;

Whereas, there are many health practices that help Christians care for their bodies and use their bodies to praise God;

Whereas, there are many health practices that foster Christian growth and learning;

Whereas, children need healthy foods and physical activity to grow, learn, and thrive;

Whereas, good health fosters faithful student attendance and quality education;

Whereas, heart disease, cancer, stroke, and diabetes are responsible for two-thirds of deaths in the United States, and major risk factors for those diseases, including unhealthy eating habits, physical inactivity, and obesity, are usually established in childhood;

Whereas, 33 percent of high school students do not participate in sufficient vigorous physical activity to maintain good health;

Whereas, only 2 percent of children (ages 2 to 19 years old) eat a healthy diet consistent with the five main recommendations of the Food Guide Pyramid;

Whereas, the most common items sold from school vending machines, school stores, and school snack bars are low-nutrition foods and beverages;

Whereas, community participation is essential to the development and implementation of successful school wellness policies;

St. Luke Lutheran School is committed to providing a school environment that promotes and protects children's health, well-being, and ability to learn by supporting healthy eating practices and rigorous physical activity for all children.

School Policy

It is the policy of St. Luke Lutheran School to

• Engage students, parents, teachers, food-service professionals, health professionals, and other interested community members in developing, implementing, monitoring, and reviewing its nutrition and physical activity policies;

• Provide opportunities, support, and encouragement to all students to be physically active on a regular basis;

• Sell or serve food and beverages that meet the nutrition recommendations of the United States Dietary Guidelines for Americans;

• Provide a variety of affordable, nutritious, and appealing foods that meet the health and nutrition needs of students;

• Employ qualified people in food-service positions who are familiar with nutrition and meal planning and preparation that promotes healthy eating;

• Provide clean, safe, and pleasant settings and adequate time for students to eat;

• Provide nutrition education and physical education to foster lifelong habits of healthy eating and physical activity; and

• Establish linkages between health education in the school, the school meal programs, and various community services.

School Goals

I. Establish a School Health Council

The Board of Parish Education will establish and work with a School Health Council to develop, implement, monitor, review, and, as necessary, revise school nutrition and physical activity policies. The School Health Council will consist of people representing the school, the congregation, the community, the school food-preparation staff, teachers, and health professionals.

St. Luke Lutheran School highly values the health and well-being of every staff member and will plan and implement activities and policies that support personal efforts by staff members to maintain a healthy lifestyle. The school supports the establishment of a staff wellness committee to develop, promote, and oversee a multifaceted plan to promote staff health and wellness. The plan should be based on input from the staff and should outline ways to encourage healthy eating, physical activity, and other aspects of a healthy lifestyle. A plan should be developed and distributed to the staff annually.

II. Sell and Serve Only Foods and Beverages of High Nutritional Quality

School meals will be appealing and attractive to children; be served in clean and pleasant surroundings; meet, at a minimum, the nutrition requirements established by local, state, and federal statutes and regulations; offer a variety of fruits and vegetables; and ensure that half of the served grains are whole grains.

St. Luke Lutheran School will involve students and parents in taste tests of new entrees and in surveys to identify new, healthful, and appealing food choices and will share information about the nutritional content of meals with parents and students via menus, a Web site, cafeteria menu board, placards, or similar materials.

To ensure that all children have breakfast, either at home or at school, in order to meet their nutritional needs and enhance their ability to learn, St. Luke Lutheran School will operate a school breakfast program if sufficient numbers of students warrant this program; arrange bus schedules and make other arrangements to encourage participation in school-served breakfasts; notify parents and students of the availability of the school breakfast program; and encourage parents to provide a healthy breakfast for their children through newsletter articles, take-home materials, or other means.

St. Luke Lutheran School will make every effort to eliminate any social stigma attached to, and prevent the overt identification of, students who are eligible for free and reduced-price school meals.

Mealtime scheduling will provide students with at least ten minutes to eat after sitting down for breakfast and twenty minutes after sitting down for lunch; schedule meal periods at appropriate times, with lunch being served between 11 a.m. and 1 p.m.; allow students to eat lunch during activities scheduled during lunch periods, including any club meetings, tutoring, or any other organizational meetings; provide students access to hand washing or sanitizing before they eat meals or snacks; and provide reasonable accommodations for toothbrushing regimens of students with special oral health needs.

To ensure that qualified people administer and operate the school food-service programs, St. Luke Lutheran School will make available continuing professional development programs for staff personnel. These programs will be appropriate to the level of responsibility involved and include certification and training programs that focus on nutrition, food preparation, and safety.

Out of concern for children who have allergies and for students who have restrictions on their diets, St. Luke Lutheran School personnel will discourage students from sharing their foods and beverages with one another during meal and snack times.

Foods and beverages offered or sold at school-sponsored events outside the school day will meet the nutrition standards for meals or for foods and beverages sold individually, as described in this policy and goal statement.

St. Luke Lutheran School will not use foods or beverages, especially those that do not meet the nutrition standards for foods and beverages sold individually, as described in this statement, as rewards for academic performance or good behavior. The school will not withhold food or beverages as a punishment.

Snacks served during the school day or in after-school care or enrichment programs will make a positive contribution to children's diets and health. These snacks will emphasize serving fruits and vegetables as the primary snack and water as the primary beverage. The school will assess if and when to offer snacks based on school mealtimes, children's nutritional needs and ages, and other considerations. A list of healthful snack items will be prepared and disseminated to teachers, after-school program personnel, and parents.

To support children's health and school nutrition-education efforts, school fund-raising activities at St. Luke Lutheran School will not involve food or will use only foods that meet the nutrition and portion size standards for foods and beverages as described in this policy statement. The school encourages fund-raising activities that promote physical activity. A list of acceptable fund-raising activities will be made available through the school office.

The administration and school food-service program of St. Luke Lutheran School will have the responsibility to approve or disapprove of all food and beverage items suggested for sale on the school campus. Food for elementary students will be made available in balanced meals. Individual food and beverage items will be limited to low-fat and nonfat milk, fruits, and nonfried vegetables. Food items offered to students, including those items made available in vending machines, a la carte lines, fund-raising activities, or in after-school programs, must meet the following nutrition and portion-size standards:

A. Permitted beverages are water or seltzer water without caloric sweeteners; fruit and vegetable juices; fruit-based drinks that contain at least 50 percent fruit juice and that do not contain caloric sweeteners; unflavored low-fat or fat-free fluid milk and nutritionally equivalent nondairy beverages, as defined by the USDA. Beverages that are not permitted are soft drinks containing caloric sweeteners; sports drinks; iced teas; fruit-based drinks that contain less than 50 percent real fruit juice or that contain caloric sweeteners; beverages containing caffeine, excluding low-fat or fat-free chocolate milk (which contain small amounts of caffeine).

B. Individually sold food items will have no more than 35 percent of the calories from fat (excluding nuts, seeds, peanut butter, and other nut butters) and 10 percent of the calories from saturated and trans fat combined; have no more than 35 percent of the weight from added sugars; contain no more than 230 milligrams of sodium per serving for chips, cereals, crackers, French fries, baked goods, and other snack items; contain no more than 480 milligrams of sodium per serving

for pastas, meats, and soups; and contain no more than 600 milligrams of sodium for pizza, sandwiches, and main dishes. A choice of at least two fruits and/or nonfried vegetables will be offered for sale at any location on the school campus where foods are sold. Items that may be included are fresh fruits and vegetables; 100 percent fruit or vegetable juices; fruit-based drinks that are at least 50 percent fruit juice and that do not contain caloric sweeteners; cooked, dried, or canned fruits (canned in fruit juice or light syrup); and cooked, dried, or canned vegetables that meet the fat and sodium guidelines.

C. Portion sizes of foods and beverages sold on the campus of St. Luke Lutheran School are limited to 1¼ ounces for chips, crackers, popcorn, cereal, trail mix, nuts, seeds, dried fruit, or jerky; 1 ounce for cookies; 2 ounces for cereal bars, granola bars, pastries, muffins, doughnuts, bagels, and other bakery items; 4 fluid ounces for frozen desserts, including low-fat or fat-free ice cream; 8 ounces of non-frozen yogurt; and 12 fluid ounces for beverages, excluding water. The portion size of a la carte entrees and side dishes, including potatoes, will not be greater than the size of comparable portions offered as part of school meals. Fruits and nonfried vegetables are exempt from portion-size limits.

III. Promote Sound Nutrition Education

St. Luke Lutheran School aims to teach, encourage, and support healthy eating by students. The school will provide nutrition education and conduct nutrition promotion activities at each grade level as part of a sequential, comprehensive, standards-based program designed to provide students with the knowledge and skills necessary to promote and protect their health. These activities are to be part of health education classes and in conjunction with classroom instruction in the various subject matter areas, as appropriate.

They are to be enjoyable, developmentally appropriate, culturally relevant, and participatory, such as contests, promotions, taste testing, farm visits, and school gardens. The content will promote fruits, vegetables, whole-grain products, low-fat and fat-free dairy products, healthy food preparation methods, and health-enhancing nutrition practices; emphasize caloric balance between food intake and energy-expending activity and exercise; and teach media literacy as it relates to food marketing. The school will provide training for teachers and staff, and link school meal programs, other school food programs, and nutritionally related community services.

School-based marketing will be consistent with nutrition education and health promotion. St. Luke Lutheran School will limit food and beverage marketing to the promotion of foods and beverages that meet the nutrition standards outlined previously in this wellness policy. School-based marketing of brands promoting predominantly low-nutrition foods and beverages is prohibited. The promotion of healthy foods, including fruits, vegetables, whole grains, and low-fat dairy products is encouraged. Examples of marketing techniques that might be used to promote nutrition education and health include vending machine covers that promote water, pricing structures that promote healthy options in a la carte lines or vending machines, sales of fruit for fundraisers, and coupons for discount gym memberships.

IV. Provide Physical Education Opportunities

At St. Luke Lutheran School, all students, including students with disabilities, special health-care needs, and in other education settings offered by the school, will receive the equivalent of 150 minutes of physical education (225 minutes in the middle school) each week for the entire school year. The school will regularly make available training in physical education for its staff and seek to maintain a certified physical education teacher on its staff as a resource person. Student involvement in other activities, such as interscholastic or intramural sports, involving physical activity will not be substituted for meeting the physical education requirement. Students will spend at least 50 percent of the physical education class time participating in moderate to vigorous physical activity.

At St. Luke Lutheran School, all elementary students will have at least twenty minutes a day of supervised recess, preferably outdoors. During this time, staff will encourage moderate to vigorous physical activity, and the school will provide safe space and equipment for this recess activity. Extended periods of inactivity on the part of students will be limited. When various school activities and weather conditions make it necessary for students to remain indoors for long periods of time, St. Luke Luthcran School will give students periodic breaks to stand and be moderately active.

St. Luke Lutheran School will offer extracurricular activity programs, such as activity clubs or intramural programs. As appropriate, interscholastic sports programs will be offered. The school will offer a range of activities that meet the needs, interests, and abilities of all students, including boys, girls, students with disabilities, and students with special health-care needs. After-school child care and enrichment programs at St. Luke Lutheran School will provide and encourage daily periods of moderate to vigorous physical activity for all participants. Space, equipment, supervision, and ideas for activities will be provided.

V. Regularly Communicate with Parents

St. Luke Lutheran School will support parents' efforts to provide a healthy diet and daily physical activity for their children. On occasion, the school in cooperation with our parents' organization (PTL) will offer healthy eating seminars for parents, send home nutrition information or post it on the school Web site, and provide nutrient analyses of school menus. At various times of the year, the school will encourage parents to pack healthy lunches and snacks and to refrain from including beverages and foods that do not meet the nutrition standards outlined in this policy. The school will provide parents with a list of foods that meet the school snack standards and provide ideas for healthy celebrations/parties, rewards, and fund-raising activities. Parents will be invited to share their healthy food practices with others in the school community.

St. Luke Lutheran School will also provide information about physical education and other school-based physical activity opportunities before, during, and after the school day and will support parents' efforts to provide children with opportunities to be physically active. Such support will include sharing information about physical activity and physical education through the school Web site, newsletter, or other take-home materials, during special events, and in physical education homework.

VI. Provide for Monitoring and Reviewing of This Wellness Policy

The principal or other designee of the Board of Education will ensure compliance with this established wellness policy and will report the school's compliance to the Board of Education at least once each year.

School food-service staff will ensure compliance with nutrition policies of the school food service and will report to the Board of Education annually regarding compliance. USDA reviews of the school lunch program will be provided to the administration and Board of Education of St. Luke Lutheran School.

To initially develop a wellness policy at St. Luke Lutheran School, a baseline assessment of exist-ing nutrition and physical activity environments and activities will be conducted. This assessment will be used to identify and prioritize improvement activities. Assessments will be repeated in conjunction with the accreditation process of St. Luke Lutheran School and the National Lutheran Schools Assessment Program. The recommendations of the Assessment Team will be reviewed and, as necessary, the wellness policy and associated activities and policies will be revised and work plans developed to facilitate implementation of the recommendations.

Discussion Questions

1. What aspects of the Model Wellness Policy are already in place in our school?

2. What aspects of the wellness policy are not in place but could be put into place with little effort?

3. What aspects of the policy are not in place and would require major effort and change of thinking?

4. What biblical statements, Christian doctrines, and worship elements could be used to foster healthy nutrition and physical activity practices among our people? Where might these statements be included in our wellness policy?

INDEX